SpringerBriefs in Psychology

For further volumes:
http://www.springer.com/series/10143

Töres Theorell

Psychological Health Effects of Musical Experiences

Theories, Studies and Reflections in Music Health Science

Springer

Töres Theorell
Karolinska Institutet
Stockholm University
Stockholm
Sweden

ISSN 2192-8363 ISSN 2192-8371 (electronic)
ISBN 978-94-017-8919-6 ISBN 978-94-017-8920-2 (eBook)
DOI 10.1007/978-94-017-8920-2
Springer Dordrecht Heidelberg New York London

Library of Congress Control Number: 2014935155

Printed on acid-free paper

Springer is part of Springer Science+Business Media (www.springer.com)

Contents

Chapter 1
Introduction

This book is about links between music and health. The emphasis is on music and public health, i.e health effects of listening to and making music in the general population. Relationships between music and health may arise in several ways. Those who have not given so much thought to this might say that music makes us relaxed and calm and that this explains why music could make us healthier. But this is not the only way in which music may influence our health. More often, we use music as a stimulant when we feel tired. Sometimes we use music for distraction. In music therapy, music is used for the release and amplification of feelings that are useful during a psychological healing process. And then, we are talking about a wide range of feelings, from pride to sadness and from joy to anger. From time to time, we all amplify different kinds of feelings by means of musical experiences even when we are not talking about music therapy. A point of departure for our thinking about music and health may be the stress concept. As we shall see, music may both increase and decrease stress. In order to create a theoretical basis for the rest of the book, I decided to devote the first chapter to the stress concept and stress mechanisms and how these relate to music in our lives.

So what role does music play in relation to our health? Let us first ask the question what role music has in modern life in general. Perhaps human beings are more exposed to music today than ever. We can see people carrying portable listening equipments in the subway, and we can hear music everywhere in homes, shops, offices and public places. The music industry is growing. But music has always been around in the history of mankind. There have even been serious scientific discussions (Mithen 2005) about the possible musical talents and activities of our ancestors the Neanderthals. According to archaeological findings, these prehistorical people have produced flutes made from bones already more than 40,000 years ago, and this means that music may have been important for them. Some authors have emphasised that music may have been important for group survival when the group was exposed to dangerous environments. Music was used along with dance and religious and other rituals in order to strengthen group cohesiveness. And cohesiveness was, for instance, important for group trust in guarding against attacks from wild animals at night (see Hagen and Bryant 2003).

T. Theorell, *Psychological Health Effects of Musical Experiences*,
SpringerBriefs in Psychology, DOI: 10.1007/978-94-017-8920-2_1,

If music has been important to the survival of the first human beings, it could also be that those who did not manage to be included in tight cohesiveness may have been less likely than others to survive. The individual willingness and ability to be included in a musical context may have been an important component here. That does not necessarily mean that those who were more likely to survive were good producers of music, but perhaps they were better listening participants—more able to experience strong musical cohesiveness—than those who did not survive? Prehistorical cave paintings in different parts of the world, produced tens of thousands of years ago, have been interpreted as pictures of ecstatic experiences. Music may have had a role in this since musical instruments appear in some of them. The social aspects of music have been important for human beings for thousands of years and remain important still today. In contemporary society, the social effects of music are utilised for commercial and political purposes. We are not always aware of this. Social aspects of music listening and production are accordingly in focus in Chap. 2. Chapter 3 focuses a specific aspect of music's social functioning namely the religious music.

The possible survival value of music has been discussed in the scientific literature. Some researchers have dismissed it. My interpretation is that the survival aspect can only be dismissed if we regard listeners and producers of music as solitary individuals only. However, if we use a group perspective, the survival value may become more obvious. There is contemporary research that makes it likely that music strengthening group cohesiveness may prolong life even today, although the mechanisms are different and not well explored. Such discussions also show how difficult it is to scientifically "isolate" the independent effect of music per se. Music is always presented in a given context (acoustics, smells, light and social environment).

To be a better music performer—to be a better instrument player or singer—than other people may not have any survival value in itself, although there are poetical descriptions of dangerous situations in which a good performer used his/her music for survival. The most famous example is the legend about Orpheus who played on his lute in order to soften the demons when he walked through the world of the dead. But, as pointed out earlier, ability to participate in musical experiences may also have a survival value. Tone deafness is very uncommon in the general population, and amusia (lack of ability to perceive that music has any meaning at all), a neurological condition, is even more infrequent. The fact that tone deafness and amusia are so uncommon may speak in favour of the opinion that ability to enjoy music has favoured survival through thousands of years.

There is a lively scientific discussion is about the possible role of music in stimulating violence and use of drugs. Some researchers have maintained that some kinds of music may have such negative effects (Sloboda and O'Neill 2001; Roberts et al. 1998) and that such music may even raise the risk of suicide (Stack and Gundlach 1992). Other researchers claim that this is not the case. The rapid distribution and the high availability of such music contribute to the importance of this since music amplifies emotions and communication between people, something that can be utilised by commercial and political forces (see for instance Brown and Theorell 2006).

Different social groups and different age groups prefer different kinds of music. This is a logical consequence of music's strong effect on group cohesion and group identity. In 1956, when I was thirteen years old, I joined my parents when they played solo parts (violin and piano) with the chamber orchestra in Kiruna, a small mining city, north of the Arctic circle in Swedish Lapland. I was allowed to participate as a temporary orchestra member. Most of the members of the orchestra were mining workers who loved classical music. I was very impressed by the joy with which they played Mozart. Later during the 1970s, this music was considered upper class music, and the mining company was forced to shut down the orchestra. This is a problematic aspect of the social stratification of music. Classical music is not in itself "upper class", but it has been associated with higher social class. People in lower social classes may find that the upper class has isolated itself socially partly by means of this music.

Rap and heavy metal are music genres that started as social protest movements for young people with small social resources. They have been subjected to sociological analysis with the central question: are they dangerous for our youth? There is no simple answer to this question. Different kinds of music have different effects and correspond to different kinds of needs. In order to make it even more complicated, different groups of researchers have had different points of departure when they have studied this question. One group of researchers (Ballard and Coates 1995), for instance, found that rap seemed to trigger more anger than did heavy metal. Another group (Rubin et al. 2001) found that heavy metal might have mirrored underlying feelings of aggression and lack of respect for women. According to Rubin et al., those who chose rap felt more aggression and less trust in other people than others. While the first group of authors emphasised the feelings that music can trigger, the other group of researchers thought that a defined type of music was chosen by a corresponding group of subjects; hence, the music genre mirrored feelings that were already there. The latter type of theory dominated the discussion during a period. One theory was that the important underlying factor could be sensation seeking. According to that hypothesis, persons with a high degree of sensation seeking were attracted by hard rock and heavy metal. They may also have been drawn to antisocial groups (Arnett 1992). However, antisocial behaviour might have been stimulated by social factors existing in specific groups. Sensation seeking is only partly inherited biologically. It is amplified or weakened by the surrounding social conditions. Therefore, the two contrasting researcher positions are not so far away from one another as one might believe. It should be pointed out that social patterns change rapidly. Therefore, it is not possible to generalise this discussion to the situation today.

Another aspect of the use of music is that it can also be used for "shutting oneself off from the community" so that we get rid of disturbing sounds in our environment. With modern portable music listening equipment, we can listen to music that people in our immediate vicinity cannot hear. This is of course the opposite of the cohesiveness aspect that I would like to discuss; people around the listener become totally unimportant, they are almost like furniture. Despite that this kind of music listening has such an antisocial aspect, there is still one remaining social component: The listener feels togetherness with those who produced the music, and the group of people who are likely to listen to it. Therefore, even that type of listening may strengthen group cohesiveness, albeit not with those who surround the listener physically for the moment.

During concentrated listening, music could serve as a distracting factor: music is used for the purpose of forgetting or "pushing out" a problem. The opposite is also frequent: if I have had a bad experience at work and I feel sad I may go home switching on some really depressing music in order to really dwell in my own sadness.

The common denominator of all these uses is that we use music for dampening, amplifying or arousing specific feelings. Others may also do this to us. I am thinking of composers of music used in films and advertisements. They are consciously manipulating our feelings when we take part in something that is not primarily musical. Most composers of such music are probably not prepared to share their knowledge with us. During earlier music periods, for instance the baroque, textbooks were produced, cookbooks telling the reader how to amplify specific types of emotional states—Affektenlehre (see Mattheson 1739).

Like, for instance, singing birds, whales and gibbon apes, music has importance also for contemporary human beings in the creation of love relationships. I am myself an example of this. Both my maternal and paternal grandparents met and fell in love when they were making music together. My paternal grandfather was singing the bass solo in Haydn's Creation when my grandmother accompanied him on the piano. And this was the start of a marital relationship. My maternal grandparents started their relationship by singing duets. I have married twice, and music was an important part in the start of both marriages. In families without active music performers, music is mostly of significance in the creation of "appropriate" emotional conditions in mating processes.

There are two personal points of departure in this book: one is my own experience of music and the other one is stress research. Since I am a researching physician and since most of my research has been focussed on stress, it is natural for me to consider cardiovascular, endocrine and immune reactions when I listen to or perform music. A considerable part of the book is accordingly based upon research that I have been doing with colleagues. It has not been so easy to find funding for research on bodily effects of music, and progress has therefore been rather slow in this field particularly when comparing with other research areas that I have been involved in. When I talk about myself and my colleagues, I am referring to a rather large group of researchers who have often been doing other kinds of research at the same time as they have been involved in music research. They are specifically mentioned in another part of the book.

My own musical background is predominantly in classical music. When I hear a piece of classical music played on violin and piano, I feel both secure and stimulated. My mother was a professional pianist and teacher of harpsichord at the college of music in Stockholm, and my father was an amateur violinist who almost became professional when he was young. This means that as a small boy I often had their music performed live in my ears when I was going to sleep. In particular, I remember a joyful fast piece for violin and piano (Humoresque, see notes) by a Swedish composer, Tor Aulin (1866–1914), and by a slow movement in a sonata in E minor for the same instruments by Emil Sjögren (1853–1918). Both of these composers had been influenced by impressionistic music and were my parents' contemporary musical heroes when they were young. I also heard my mother practice endlessly some of the most difficult passages in the piano part in Schubert's trout quintet. This kind of repetition became part of my feeling of security. Musical guests were frequent and chamber music was often played, for instance Johannes Brahms' trios for piano, violin and cello and Robert Schumann's quartet in E flat major for piano, violin, viola and cello. Every time I hear tunes from these pieces, I have a very special feeling of attachment.

It is likely that I heard this music even before I was born. It has been shown that the foetus is able to hear music during the third semester of the pregnancy and that after birth it reacts physiologically in specific ways to the music pieces that it has been exposed to before birth. Perhaps this could explain the special role that these pieces have for my musical experience.

Both as a child and as an adult, I have been singing and playing the violin. This has become so important for me that I cannot abstain from making music. This strong drive to perform music is of course not unique to me. The question is how it arises.

There is in me, like in everybody else, a mixture of aesthetic, emotional, social and bodily components in the experience of music. These will be further discussed in the following chapter on stress. The first component is related to aesthetic and emotional experiences. Strong musical experiences, as mentioned above, may trigger or amplify specific emotions, for instance intensive sadness, in unexpected ways. As an adult, I have almost never wept. I can only recollect one occasion on which I wept intensively. This was at my father's funeral. As long as the funeral was based upon words, I had no strong emotional reactions. However, suddenly musicians started to play the slow movement in Schubert's string quartet behind my back—a piece that I had heard my father play many times. I was emotionally unprepared for the strong effect when I started weeping strongly. The surprise effect was overwhelming since I had not seen the musicians before they started playing. Le Doux (1998) introduced the electrical "short cut" of music directly to the emotional brain. This means that the electrical music impulses are transmitted to the thalamus in the midbrain, a station for sorting all sorts of incoming signals. From the thalamus, the impulses are transmitted directly and rapidly to the emotional brain—the "lower" and more rapid path. A "higher" and slower path take impulses to the intellectual parts of the cortex. Accordingly, the emotions are much faster than the intellect in processing music. This creates an important basis for surprise effects—with emotions aroused or amplified by the music, sometimes forcing the intellect in the direction of reorientation (see chapter on treatment). Another important point is that the same piece of music does not trigger my weeping in other contexts, it was the combination of music, the specific circumstances and the memory of my father playing it that triggered the reaction.

My special need for performing music, despite the fact that I am not a professional musician, could be regarded partly as a compensatory mechanism. I do not normally express strong feelings in words in my daily life. Perhaps I share with many others the need to express feelings musically when we do not express them so easily in words? The music is needed as an "emotion loudspeaker".

Another component in the "drive to perform music" is embedded in the strong social experiences arising when we make music together. Already when we listen together to a concert, we may have such feelings of cohesiveness in relation to the other ones in the audience, but this is stronger when we form a group performing music. This togetherness has both an intellectual and an emotional part. To make music is to a great extent to find the right notes and the right rhythm. When the music is complicated, this is intellectually demanding; and when we do it together, there is a social pressure with negative as well as positive connotations. If I perform wrongly, the others may become angry with me because everyone has to repeat the part that went wrong. However, when it finally works, there may be a strong collective reward. Such reward feelings are usually stronger when there is a group performing than when the performer is performing on his or her own. If there is an audience, this adds further to the reward.

For me the collective feeling, for instance, when I have been a choral singer in Bach's passions during Easter has been very strong. In such situations, I may feel that I leave myself, becoming part of a large community. This feeling is not particularly strongly religious for me personally and reminds me of the fact that these passions are staging strong feelings that everybody can experience—mourning, hatred and pity just to name a few. "Leaving oneself" in this situation is a kind of depersonalisation. This has been described in strong musical experiences by several authors, for instance Benzon (2001, see the chapter on social aspects).

Observations of depersonalisation remind us of mysticism and religion that we shall discuss in the chapter on religious music.

In the total experience of music, there are also other kinds of sensory input. My strong need to sing may have arisen partly in my childhood when as a child I was asked to sing a Christmas song to an audience of adults. This was in a marble room with strong echoing acoustics. The physical vibrations arising in my body in this situation made an inextinguishable lifelong impression on me. Physical vibrations may also be an important component for the younger generations. It could explain why young people often want maximal volume when they listen to or perform music. Apart from such physical external sensations, there are also bodily effects of singing on the immune and endocrine systems, bodily effects that arise internally because of the external stimuli.

For all music performers, amateurs as well as professionals, the strongest reward is the "flow" feeling. This is the elated feeling of "effortless attention" which arises when after long-lasting practice, the performer manages to make music in such a way that he or she feels very content with the performance (Csikszentmihalyi 1974). There is a high arousal level. This basic feeling is something that all musicians are striving to experience. I have been fortunate enough to experience it myself several times. According to my own experiences, it may arise in many different circumstances. It does not seem to make any difference if I sing or play, if I sing alone or in a small ensemble or a big orchestra or choir. Genre does not make any difference. I have experienced it during performance of pop music, jazz and classical music. Flow is a profound phenomenon that we all want to experience. There is an element of cohesiveness with emotional undercurrent in it.

For me, the classical music has a special positive position; whereas for others, classical music may arouse negative feelings and anger. "Wrong music" in a given situation (for instance joyful dance music at a funeral) could trigger strong negative emotions. The performance of the music is also important. For instance, if Bach's Air is being played in too fast, a tempo all the calming effect gets lost. Accordingly, the emotional effects of music are determined not only by its contents but also by the performance itself, by circumstances and by previous experiences of the same or similar music. Chap. 4 in this book discusses individual physiological and psychological effects of music listening. Neurobiological aspects are, however, covered more comprehensively in other books.

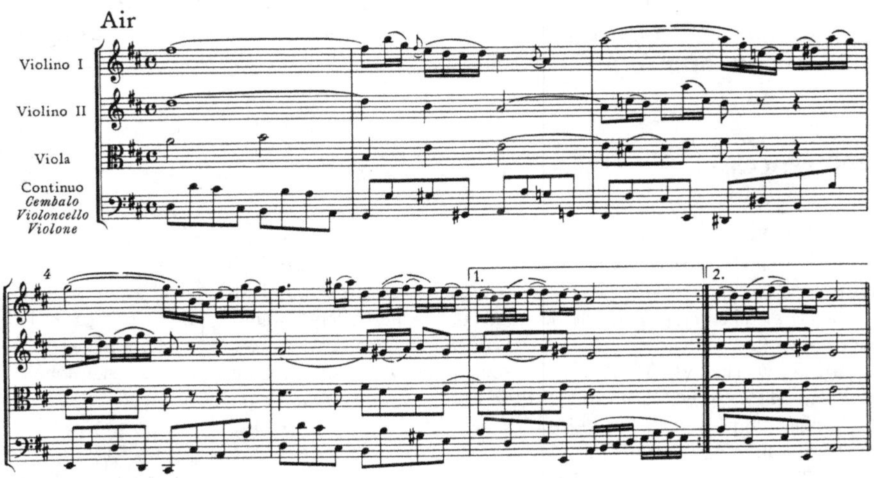

How is music used in various kinds of therapy? There is no doubt that music, if used in appropriate ways, may have beneficial effects particularly in conditions with pain and mental ill health. The fifth chapter is devoted to a discussion regarding these aspects. In this chapter, there will also be a discussion regarding possible therapeutic effects of performing music, since music therapy uses music both "passively" (listening to) and "actively" (performing). By understanding basic principles in therapy, it will also be easier for us to understand how music affects us outside therapeutic situations.

Chapter 6 deals with biological effects of a special kind of music performance, namely singing, that most people get into contact with. The seventh chapter is devoted to singing together or choral singing.

The Chap. 8 is about music in child rearing. Music could be regarded as a good tool in the development of emotions. Perhaps this is the most important use of music?

In the Chap. 9, I discuss the significance of music for musicians and their health. At a first glance, one might think that musicians should be healthier than everybody else because of the potentially good health effects of music. But first of all—as pointed out previously—all music effects are not positive, there are many situations in which music may make us feel bad. Secondly, there is a pronounced difference between living with music for joy and to earn one's living from making music. In the latter situation, performance anxiety may become a factor that affects health adversely.

Since the book covers wide areas of research, it is impossible to give reference to all the relevant literature. The reader will have to excuse me for having selected only part of the scientific references. In addition, I find it important to go into detail in some of the research in order to make it possible for the reader to become analytically critical. Since I know the research that I have been involved in myself better than other research, there is an unfair and perhaps myopic emphasis on "my" research.

The main focus in this book is on musical effects on health and their significance in society. In order to discuss this meaningfully, one has to start discussing adverse stress and how that may relate to musical experiences. Accordingly, the main question in this chapter is in what ways might music protect us against adverse effects of stress?

References

Arnett, J. (1992). The soundtrack of recklessness: musical preferences and reckless behavior among adolescents. *Journal of Adolescent Research, 7*, 313–331. doi:10.1177/074355489273003.

Ballard, M. E., & Coates, S. (1995). The immediate effects of homicidal, suicidal and nonviolent heavy metal and rap songs on the moods of college students. *Youth and Society, 27*, 148–168.

Benzon, W. (2001). *Beethoven's anvil: Music in mind and culture*. New York: Basic Books.

Brown, S., & Theorell, T. (2006). The social uses of background music for personal enhancement. In S. Brown & U. Volgsten (Eds.), *Music and manipulation: On the social uses and social control of music* (pp. 126–160). New York: Berghahn Books.

Csikszentmihalyi, M. (1974). *Beyond boredom and anxiety*. San Francisco: Jossey-Bass.

Hagen, E. H., & Bryant, G. A. (2003). Music and dance as a coalition signaling system. *Human Nature, 14*, 21–51.

Le Doux, J. (1998). *The emotional brain*. New York: Weidenfeld and Nicolson.

Mattheson, J. (1739). *Der vollkommene Kapellmeister*. Herold, Hamburg.

Mithen, S. (2005). *The singing Neanderthals: The origins of music, language, mind and body*. London: Weidenfeld and Nicholson.

Roberts, K. R., Dimsdale, J., East, P., & Friedman, L. (1998). Adolescent emotional response to music and its relationship to risk-taking behaviors. *Journal of Adolescent Health, 23*, 49–54.

Rubin, A. M., West, D. V., & Mitchell, W. S. (2001). Differences in aggression, attitudes toward women and distrust as reflected in popular music preferences. *Media Psychology, 3*, 25–42.

Sloboda, J. A., & O'Neill, S. A. (2001). Emotions in everyday listening to music. In P. N. Juslin & J. A. Sloboda (Eds.), *Music and emotion: theory and research* (pp. 415–429). Oxford: Oxford Univ. Press.

Stack, S., & Gundlach, J. H. (1992). The effect of country music on suicide. *Social Forces, 71*(1), 211–218.

Chapter 2
Stress and Music

Concepts and Mechanisms

Are there any theories that could explain why repeated exposure to music (or cultural experiences in more general terms) might influence our health? A common statement is that music is good for our health because it helps us relax. This might benefit health in some situations, but such simplistic explanations can only explain part of the potential health promotion effects of music. I do not think that modern man uses music mainly for relaxation purposes. Perhaps even quite to the contrary, in our modern era with emphasis on alertness, music is more often used as a central stimulant. In the chapter on individual singing, I will show that most people who sing regularly become both more relaxed and more alert after singing. This may seem like a paradox and does not fit the idea that most people may have about stress.

However, despite these reservations, let us start with the relaxing effect of music that many people have experienced. How does it influence health? If some kinds of music do reduce the feeling of stress in some situations, this might have a salutogenic effect (increasing positive factors) and also reduce adverse health effects of stress (decreasing negative factors). In order to discuss this, I have to introduce some basic concepts related to stress. If we do not decide what we are talking about when we talk about stress, the discussion will be confusing.

In physiology and medicine, the most frequent definition of stress is the one introduced by Selye (1956). According to Selye, *stress is a general activation reaction to a stimulus that could mean both a challenge (in a positive sense) and a threat (in a negative sense).* The activation takes place because the body needs energy in order to manage the challenge or threat. Selye was discussing that of individuals of course react differently to the same stimulus, and that different stimuli induce different mobilisation reactions. But, still according to Selye, there is a common denominator in this mobilisation reaction and arousal. That common denominator is what he labelled stress. As we shall see in coming chapters, musical experiences can both reduce and amplify stress reactions. And this frequently occurs in real-life situations.

T. Theorell, *Psychological Health Effects of Musical Experiences*, SpringerBriefs in Psychology, DOI: 10.1007/978-94-017-8920-2_2,

The importance of the surrounding factors is great, and this also means that it is difficult to isolate the "musical effect" on stress from other influences in real-life situations as well as from the influence of previous experiences with the same music.

Selye also applied a time perspective to the stress reaction with three phases, the *General Adaptation Syndrome*. The initial phase (arousal) is so rapid that the individual is not conscious of what happens—all of a sudden the body is mobilised without cognitive analysis. In the second phase (defence), the body prepares itself for fight in several ways (see below). In the third phase (exhaustion), if the stress situation lasts for a long time, the body is exhausted and not able to handle the situation as effectively as in the previous phases.

There is an intricate interplay between genes and environment when the type and intensity of the stress reaction is determined. In every moment, our biological programme determines how we react to a piece of music that we hear. The biological programme has been modelled by the experiences we have had previously in life and how they have interacted with our genes. This interaction means that some stress-related genes—for instance those who influence blood pressure elevation or activation of the immune system—become "activated". This could mean that if one is forced to listen for a long time and continuously to a disliked piece of music, such stress-related genes become activated, resulting in amplified and more frequent biological stress reactions to this piece. Interestingly, however, there is also a corresponding positive possibility, the same genes can be deactivated by pleasant music! Activation and deactivation of genes are a relatively new scientific discipline, epigenetics. Even the chemical reactions mediating such processes are now being explored, and one powerful chemical tool is methylation and demethylation of genes (Szyf 2012). If we want music to have an influence also during other life situations (without music), we would require these music-related epigenetic mechanisms to spread to life in general and to be long lasting. This is, however, merely speculation. Epigenetics is a new research field.

Figure 2.1 summarises my thoughts about the interplay between individual and environment in the experience of music. There are always a number of stressors in the environment. These will be handled by the individual programme that is constantly changing as a consequence of gene–environment interactions. The musical stimuli are located to the left in the diagram. Every time we hear a piece of music, our biological programme will respond to it, resulting in behavioural (dancing, singing, drinking, eating etc.), psychological (sad, joyful, anxious etc.) and biological (hormonal, cardiovascular, immunological etc.) reactions. Behavioural, psychological and physiological reactions are mixed with one another. We are aware of some of these reactions, but we are also unaware of many of them. Professional musicians and dancers have trained their consciousness regarding what goes on in their mind and body when they listen to or perform music or movements. All reactions, also those that we are unaware of, are stored in the box labelled "previous experiences". This could be regarded as a log book feeding our individual programme with impulses that constantly model the programme in order to make it adapted to our future music environment. The genes also contribute to the changes, but they do this in constant interaction with the musical experiences that we have in our life.

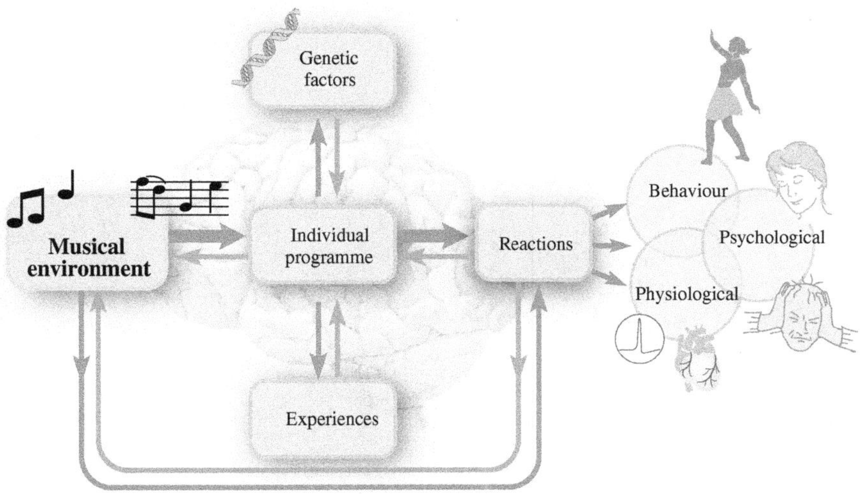

Fig. 2.1 Our biological programme. Every time we hear a piece of music, our individual programme responds behaviourally, psychologically and physiologically. These different kinds of reactions are mixed together. Genetic factors interact with our experiences. The connections are bidirectional. Some impulses influence the reactions without being an essential part of the music programme (such as vibrations). *Source* A. R. Kagan, L. Levi, T. Theorell

It is important to acknowledge that the lines between the boxes are bidirectional. Another important point is that some impulses related to the total experience but not directly music-related (such as vibrations and painfully loud sounds) can give rise to direct effects without passing the musical brain and the individual musical programme. Such processes, although they do not belong to the musical experience per se, could have strong effects on the individual's music programming.

All these reactions are stored together with the musical experience in the individual programme. This means that the reaction to the same piece will not be exactly the same when the individual gets exposed to it on subsequent occasions. Obviously, in addition, the reactions themselves may influence the musical environment. Perhaps the listener shouts aggressively at the person playing the music with the result that the music stops. If the listener shows enthusiasm, the music performance may be intensified.

The goal of the stress reaction is to prepare the body for mental and physical effort in conjunction with the challenge or threat. Energy mobilisation has the highest priority, and this means that fuel has to be provided for the expected energy-requiring work. This corresponds to increased blood concentration of free fatty acids and glucose. There are also a number of parallel effects that are important for the body in this situation, particularly if the situation is going to last for long. For instance, it is important to be insensitive to pain—if fighting leads to injury, the fighter should be able to disregard pain and continue fighting for as long as possible. For the same reason, blood coagulation is stimulated during acute stress—excessive

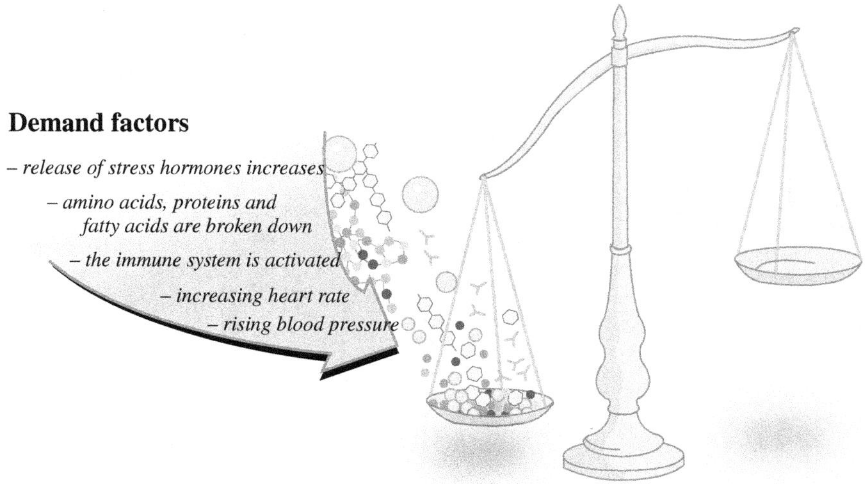

Picture 2.2 Negative stress. When the body is exposed to demands in everyday life, it is mobilising energy in order to manage the situation. Repeated such reactions without periods of rest can result in harmful processes, which are threatening the inner environment of the body. The mobilisation of energy becomes a threat. © Annika Röhl

bleeding should not weaken the body during the acute stress situation. In the same vein, some aspects of the inflammatory responses are weakened; swollen knees or muscles should not inhibit action. These types of reactions are phylogenetic which means that they have been inherited from lower animals and were of importance to the survival of human beings in the early history of mankind (Picture 2.2).

This way of reasoning can be applied directly to the use of music in the history of mankind. During wars, music has been used for arousal purposes—to increase the mobilisation of energy. The association between "strong" marches and aggression and hostile energy is evident. In line with my previous reasoning, soldiers should also not be disturbed by pain and bleeding. Research will be described in subsequent chapters illustrating that these kinds of reactions can be strengthened by aggressive war music.

We are mostly not aware of our bodily reactions to music, and accordingly, we may be unaware of the arousal effect—as adults, we have been taught to neglect it. Children are different. We had a very clear illustration of this in my family when we attended a performance of very old African war dances. As adults, we looked at this intellectually without awareness of any emotional reactions. Our three-year-old son, however, was very frightened. He reacted openly with fear—which is what these dances were intended to evoke. We were indeed looking at war dances, but we saw them merely as interesting cultural manifestations.

An additional concept is needed in the understanding of health effects of music. This relates to the bodys capacity to restore and protect itself against adverse effects of stress.

Anabolism or Regeneration

Anabolism or regeneration refers to processes that stimulate the synthesis of proteins. This is central to restoration and growth of cells. Mobilisation of energy that was described above is partly in opposition to restoration and growth of cells. Intensive mobilisation of energy is associated with downplaying of anabolism and regeneration. This creates no problem when the stress periods are short. But anabolism cannot have low priority for long periods, because vulnerability to disease increases. The organ systems become fragile because there is constant break down of cells in the body, even during days when we are not making any efforts, so called programmed cell death (Horvitz 2003). These have to replaced or repaired in anabolic activity. Conversely, if it is possible to stimulate anabolism by means of musical experiences, this could protect us against adverse effects of stress (Picture 2.3).

The basic discussion regarding stress concepts can be applied to the analysis of musical effects on health. Music may amplify feelings that we have, and it may also induce strong feelings. Thus, music can both accelerate and slow down processes in the body. Accordingly, it is no surprise that music can influence a wide range of bodily functions. So far I have discussed stress mainly in terms of biological functions. Psychological processes are parallel to bodily processes, however. The Swedish psychoanalyst Thorsten Sjöwall (1991) discussed psychological processes from a psychosomatic perspective. He used the same terminology as I have been using for the biological processes. He summarises by saying that the psyche, exactly like the body, thrives best when periods of energy mobilisation are interspersed by periods of anabolism.

In psychology, the counterpart of biological individual programme is *coping*. This is a very central concept in psychology and psychological stress research. It could be translated into "mastering problems". Active coping entails an expectation that the individual's acts will result in an improvement in the problematic situation. Listening to and performing music could influence coping in several ways, for example by infusing energy so that the individual gets the strength to deal with a problem or by facilitating new ways of thinking.

The health promoting effects we might get from regular, repeated musical experiences in everyday life could accordingly arise in three ways:

1. Inhibition of intensity and frequency of arousal reactions—music as a filter
2. Strengthening of anabolism/regeneration improving resilience in general
3. Improved coping patterns—New ways of thinking may lead to more positive expectations of successful coping.

The first mechanism implies that repeated musical experiences inducing a relaxed state occur so often that it causes a total reduction in aroused state over longer periods. This might be similar to the effects observed after periods of repeated meditation over longer periods. We know that this may induce long-lasting changes in the brain related to a lowered level of sympathetic arousal.

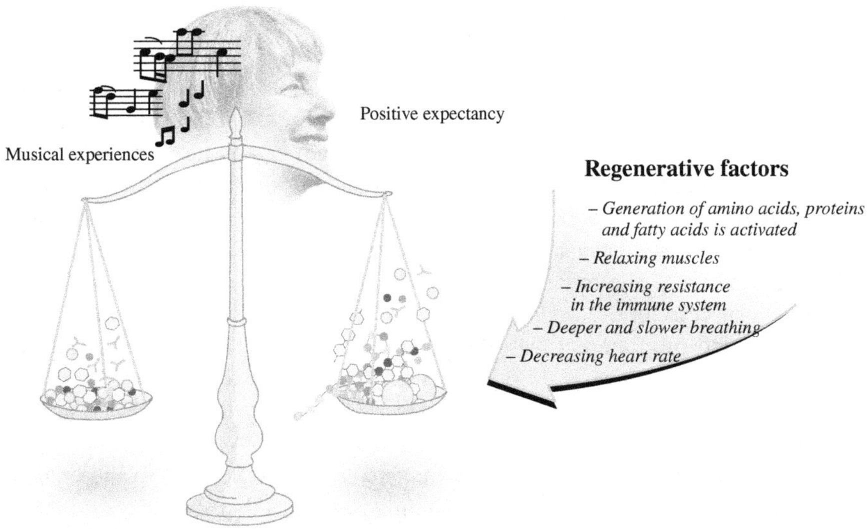

Picture 2.3 Health promoting effects. The balance can be resumed by strengthened regenerative processes. Repeated musical experiences can protect the body against harmful effects of repeated long-lasting demands. © Annika Röhl

The relaxation aspect of music is being exploited by a whole industry producing relaxing music.

The second mechanism is similar to the one operating in regular physical training, which is known to stimulate hormones that increase the body's ability to restore, repair and replace worn-out cells. Such processes have not been extensively studied in relation to musical experiences, but in the chapter about choir singing, a long-term experiment will be described, which examines the possible effect of singing in a choir on the production of a regenerative hormone.

The third mechanism has been discussed extensively in qualitative studies. For instance Gabrielsson (2011) has described strong musical experiences in 900 interviews. These interviews illustrate that strong musical experiences can change an individual's way of thinking about himself/herself dramatically and that this could change the life course. This will be discussed more extensively in the chapter about treatment. Another illustration is an experiment that was performed in northern Sweden (Bygren et al. 2009). Caregivers were offered the possibility to participate in a cultural activity experiment for employees. They were randomly allocated to either a control group or an experimental group. In the experimental group, the subjects were asked to participate in cultural activities once a week. They could choose activity from a menu including cinema, concerts, art exhibitions and choral singing. The activities took place once a week during two months. In the control group, the subjects had to wait until after the experimental period before they were allowed to take part in the cultural activities. The participants in both groups were asked to fill in a questionnaire before and after the two months that the study lasted. The results showed that those who had participated in the cultural activities felt better physically and socially, and they also reported increased vitality during the study period. The design of that study does not allow us to draw any conclusions regarding specific effects of choral singing. The beneficial development in the experimental group was statistically significantly different from that in the control group where no such changes were recorded. In this case, one might say that the third mechanism has been operating—thinking along new lines.

The third mechanism implies that expectations for successful coping in stressful situations are improved. This requires that the cultural experience makes the subject re-evaluate important aspects of life and makes him or her feel that life can be reorganised. This is the basic thinking also behind music therapy. But it is also a fundamental aspect in the use of other cultural activities in the treatment of psychological states caused by traumatic events. The most extensively studied cultural activity from this point of view is creative writing. Pennebaker (1997) and Lumley et al. (2002) have described the therapeutic processes that start when subjects are allowed to spend one week under supervision writing about their own traumatic event(s). Such research has shown that the psychological state improves in most of the subjects and that immunological and other biological beneficial changes are also likely to take place. These only last for a couple of months, however, if no follow-up takes place.

If a cultural activity has a beneficial effect on a group of subjects, there may also be secondary effects on other individuals who interact with them. This has recently been shown in an evaluation of the use of an art intervention designed to increase empathy in middle managers. The intervention lasted for nine months, with group sessions once a month. Each session contained poetry reading with themes related to ethical and moral responsibility in crisis situations. The poems were interspersed with music that was selected specifically in order to amplify emotions or to support the participants emotionally. After each session, there were group discussions and in addition reactions were followed up in diaries. The evaluation was performed as a random-controlled study, which means that half of the studied managers were allocated to the art intervention and half of them to a more conventionally designed high-quality education programme with lectures and subsequent group discussions (Romanowska et al. 2011). Follow-up 18 months after start of the employees working for the managers in the two groups showed that the art intervention had been more successful than the other intervention. This was reflected among other things in a more beneficial development of the regenerative hormone DHEA-s in the employees working for the managers in the art intervention group. Thus, it is possible that a mixture of poetry and music may influence not only the listeners themselves but also their subordinates.

In later chapters, I shall describe more in detail how the two first mechanisms (reduction in arousal and stimulation of anabolism/regeneration) might explain health effects of music. In Chap. 3, I shall discuss how music influences social interactions.

References

Bygren, L. O., Weissglas, G., Wikström, B. M., Konlaan, B. B., Grjibovski, A., Karlsson, A. B., et al. (2009). Cultural participation and health: a randomized controlled trial among medical care staff. *Psychosomatic Medicine, 71*, 469–473.

Gabrielsson, A. (2011). *Strong experiences with music: Music is much more than just music*. Oxford: Oxford University Press.

Horvitz HR (2003) Worms, life and death (Nobel lecture)—review. *ChemBiochem* 697–711.

Lumley, M. A., Tojek, T.M., & Macklem, D.J. (2002). Effects of written emotional disclosure among repressive and alexithymic people. In S. J. Lepore & J. M. Smyth (Eds.), *The writing cure: How expressive writing promotes health and emotional well-being*. Washington DC: American Psychological Association.

Pennebaker, J. (1997). Writing about emotional experiences as a therapeutic process. *Psychological Science, 8*, 162–166.

Romanowska, J., Larsson, G., Eriksson, M., Wikström, B.-M., Westerlund, H., & Theorell, T. (2011). Health effects on leaders and co-workers of an art-based leadership development program. *Psychotherapy and Psychosomatics, 80*, 78–87.

Selye, H. (1956). *The stress of life*. New York: McGraw-Hill. ISBN 978-0070562127.

Sjöwall, T. (1991). Psykosomatiska grundbegrepp (Psychosomatic basics). In J. K. Konarski-Svensson & T. Theorell (Eds.), *Psykosomatisk läkekonst (Psychosomatic medicine)*. Stockholm: Natur & Kultur Förlaget.

Szyf, M. (2012). Mind-body interrelationship in DNA methylation. *Chemical Immunology and Allergy, 98*, 85–99.

Chapter 3
Music in Social Cohesion

Social Support as a Health Promoting Factor

What I have discussed so far points at the importance of musical activity as a factor promoting a group's cohesiveness. Maybe this is the most important aspect of musical activity in health promotion. Group cohesion has been shown to be a health promoting factor in itself, not only in ancient history when the everyday environment was quite dangerous physically and group cohesiveness could protect against violent death (Berg 2005), but also for modern man facing symbolic threats. Good social support has been shown to protect against premature cardiac death, for instance. But what is the nature of this social effect of music?

The American jazz musician and social anthropologist Benzon (2001) has stated that music is the most effective social *tool for brain coupling* that man has invented. When I saw that formulation, I found it fantastic as an image of the social power of music. I imagined 10,000 people at a rock concert or another 10,000 singing opera choirs with Luciano Pavarotti as their soloist. Of course, people who take part in such events have a very strong feeling of cohesiveness. The rhythm is exactly the same for all the participants although other aspects of the music experience are flavoured by previous experiences. You can almost see the rhythmic waves going between the brains of all these people. Public health work has been increasingly influenced by this insight. For instance, choir singing open to everybody has become increasingly successful as part of public health promotion work in England (Clift 2012) (see the chapter on individual singing).

As expected, slow deep breathing occurs when singers perform unison, well structured wordless songs with long phrases. This breathing pattern is related to variations in heart rate, which slows down during exhalation and speeds up during inhalation. Such variations may occur in a coordinated way in choir singers (Vickhoff et al. 2013). Breathing and heart rate effects are the same as those arising when

This chapter was preceded by a large two-page picture (page 24–25), showing a Swedish composer/conductor Alfvén who conducts 10,000 Swedish male choir singers in 1923.

T. Theorell, *Psychological Health Effects of Musical Experiences*,
SpringerBriefs in Psychology, DOI: 10.1007/978-94-017-8920-2_3,

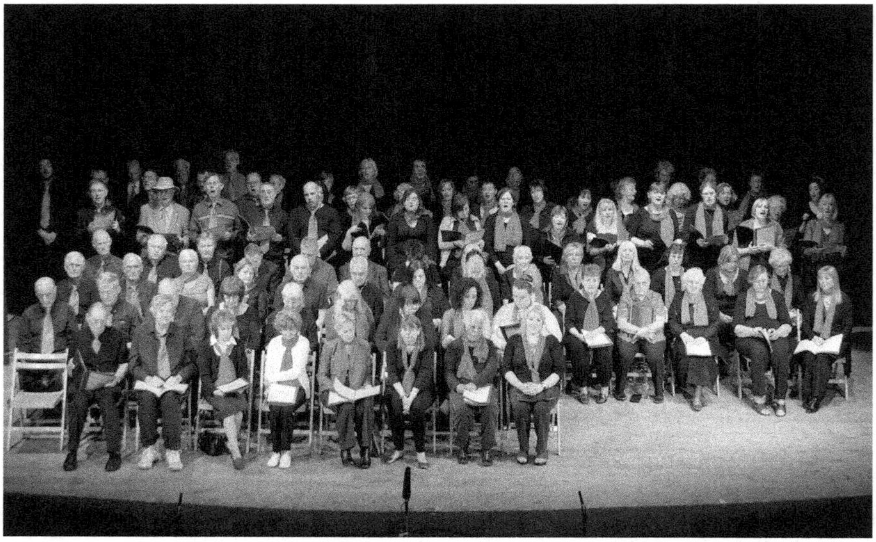

Picture 3.1 Choir for rehabilitation in Folkstone, England. Courtesy of Stephen Clift

we say manthras, for instance the difference of course being that the song in itself strengthens the possibility for the participants to follow the rhythm. The music provides a strong motivation for joint breathing cycles. When more complicated songs are performed and when the singers sing in different voices (soprano, alto, tenor and bass), this strong coordination is likely to disappear. When words are added to the sound, the psychophysiological patterns become even more complicated (Olsson et al. 2013). Following this reasoning, slow, unison, wordless singing (or singing with few simple words) may be of particular importance to group cohesiveness. But, of course, more complicated choir singing may be very powerful in triggering joint strong emotions despite individual differences in physiological phase.

Choir singing is also being evaluated scientifically as a means of curing depression and burnout syndrome. Picture 3.1 shows the members of a choir for patients with such diagnoses. Clinical experiences with choral singing activities occurring regularly over several months tell us that the participants can gain assertiveness and health benefits (the picture is shown with courtesy of Stephen Clift, Canterbury University, Institute for Arts and Health, Folkestone).

An interesting biological background behind the collective effect of music was discovered when "mirror neurons" were found. When we see a person perform an act that we often perform ourselves and that we can identify us with, those parts of the brain that order us to perform the same act are activated despite the fact that we actually do not perform the act. Studies of the brain activation in a pianist listening to a recording of a piece that he/she has played show that those brain areas commanding the fingers that should do the job are activated in a very precise manner. In addition, the brain activation precedes the music. If the notes in the music demands that the left fifth finger presses a given key on the piano, the corresponding "motor" area of the brain is

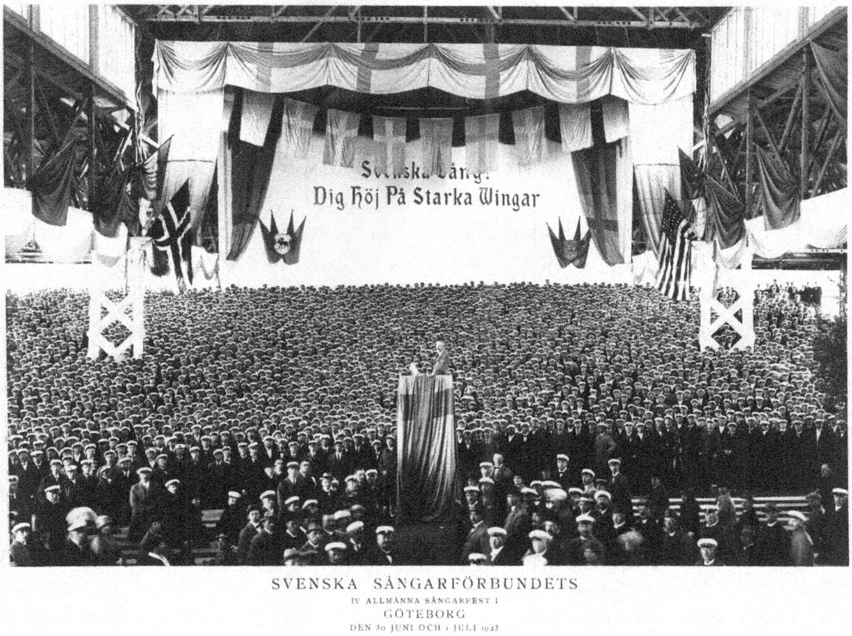
Dig Höj På Starka Wingar
SVENSKA SÅNGARFÖRBUNDETS
IV ALLMÄNNA SÅNGARFEST I
GÖTEBORG
DEN 30 JUNI OCH 1 JULI 1923

Picture 3.2 Male Choir

electrically activated 300 ms before the sound is heard in the recording. When we hear music, if we have experienced or performed this particular piece of music previously, there is accordingly an activation not only of the parts of the brain that are associated with the listening but also those parts that are associated with performing. This will differ depending on the listener, whether he or she is a music performer or not, and also on whether he or she is acquainted with the music or not (Vickhoff 2008).

Large gatherings of thousands of people experience music together in our time. This is an old tradition. Picture 3.2 shows a gathering of male choir singers singing together in Göteborg, Sweden, in 1923. They represent a prevalent Nordic form of choir singing during these years. The conductor on the picture is the well-known composer Hugo Alfvén. Choir festivals for large numbers of people from the world are organised more and more frequently around the world today. It is felt that this could strengthen the collaboration between countries (see, for instance de Quadros and Dorstewitz 2011). Such large choirs have not existed in mankind's long early history, which has been the basis of genetic selection. But dancing and rhythmic sound may have increased the cohesiveness in small groups. Mithen (2005) has developed a theory regarding Neanderthalers making music. This theory has been based upon archaeological findings of primitive music instruments that have are likely to have been produced by these prehistorical human beings. Dance, music and religious rituals have probably been created in an early stage of history for the stimulation of cohesiveness. If the cohesiveness is strong, the members of the group can trust one another when they take turns to watch for dangerous enemies day and night. This increases the likelihood of survival in our ancestors' environment that was full of threats. The more effective these methods for increased cohesiveness have been, the greater the longevity. Conversely, those individuals who have not been able to relate to music may have had shorter longevity. Accordingly, musicality or at least ability to relate socially to group music may have benefitted genetic selection during tens of thousands of years. What speaks in favour of this theory is that subjects who lack musicality are so infrequent. This may surprise the reader since we often hear the statement: "I lack musicality". Most of the subjects who say so, however, lack musical training but may actually have a potential for developing their musicality. Sacks (2007) has summarised this by saying that approximately 5 % of the normal population are tone deaf. Tone deafness is inability to differentiate intervals (which is the higher note when two notes are being played?). But even, those 5 % tone deaf mostly appreciate music and are able to relate to it. Even fewer suffer from amusia, an extremely infrequent neurological condition, which Sacks has also described. Amusia means that it is impossible to understand musical sound as in any way meaningful. A concert is always a painful experience to such a person.

Animals also sing. For them, singing often have an obvious social meaning. First of all, I am thinking of birds. The male bird singing is often a very important factor in the attraction of females. Singing plays an important role in the life of our close relative the gibbon ape (Brown 2000), and in that species the ability to sing plays an important role in the female's selection of partner. Once a gibbon pair has been established, the female and male stay in fidelity throughout the rest of their lives, and singing remains an important part of their lives.

Theories have been developed regarding the motifs of the 10,000 to 30,000-years-old cave paintings (Altamira, Chauvet, Lascaux) that have been found in several European countries (France, Italy, Spain, Portugal, Ireland, see Berg 2005). The animal motifs have drawn the most attention, but there are a great deal of illustrations showing extatic group experiences that may have contained musical experiences. These paintings are strikingly similar despite the fact that the geographical and temporal distances between them are enormous. One interpretation of this is that these kinds of extatic group experiences are of fundamental importance to all human beings. Our biology is constructed for periods of arousal, and effort interspersed with periods of relaxation and recuperation. The most obvious example known to most people is how muscles are kept in shape. The muscles are built up when we rest but the process is inhibited if do not allow ourselves to relax between the periods of effort. The regenerative anabolic hormones that build up our muscles are in their most active phase when we rest, but they need guidance from the efforts in order to know how to build up the muscles. Humans who lived a very long time ago may have had boring passive periods, e.g. during the dark winters living in caves. They may have needed extatic explosions now and then for their well-being. The ecstasy may also have been important for mating and family formation. As I mentioned before, such gatherings with dancing and music, as well as the paintings documenting them, may have been important for group cohesiveness.

The Norwegian music researcher Björkvold (2005) has pointed out that spontaneous children's songs in the USA, Scandinavia and Russia have common archaic traits and that this is still true today despite the massive influence on children of television and other modern media. A simple example is the short phrase below that seems to exist in many languages.

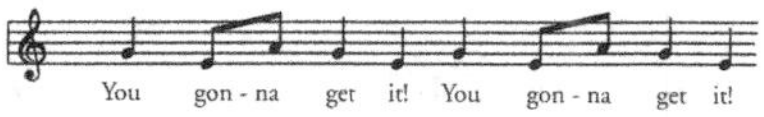

Phrases like this have existed in many cultures long before the introduction of television and other modern forms of sound communication. It could be hypothesised that a massive massmedia exposure to adult music ought to distract children from such spontaneous children's songs but they seem to resist this type of influence. That spontaneous children's songs in their original forms are still existing might be explained by common basic culture for all humans. Another way of looking at it would be to say that spontaneous music making is programmed in human beings.

In a dramatic case description, Sacks (2007) has illustrated that music may be more programmed in our brains than most of us would believe. He is describing what happened to Tony Cicoria, a 42-year-old orthopaedic surgeon who was hit one day by a thunder flash. He was unconscious for several days. During a long-period afterwards, he had memory problems that finally disappeared so that he was able to start working normally as a surgeon again. After waking up, however, it turned out that he all of a sudden was passionately interested in music, which he had not been previously. As a child, he had played a little piano but found it uninteresting. Now, however, he had an incessant need to play the piano and to compose. This filled all of his leisure time. One is tempted to think in such a case that the flash had cut-off some inhibition in his brain—something that liberated his strong interest in music.

There are also descriptions of subjects with serious neurological handicaps, showing extremely well-developed musicality. The most famous example is Mozart. There is relatively strong evidence that Mozart suffered from Tourette's syndrome (Simkin 1992), a neurological disorder with compulsive movements, vocalisations and poor ability to control statements. Tourette patients lack part of the impulse inhibition that most of us have and which makes us function well socially. But instead, many of these patients have developed extreme musical talents. Sacks describes among other cases a pianist and a drummer. Although the Tourette patients experience difficulties in their social contacts, the example may show that if some inhibitions would be removed many of us would turn out to have much stronger musical talents than we know. The strong musicality that may be partly hidden in us may have been more important in earlier phases of mankind's history. Today, we are inhibiting it more than we stimulate it. There are many descriptions from early school experiences. Many boys and girls were told that they were unable to sing and were not even allowed to participate in the music lessons. I have heard many such stories, with deep sadness reactions. Men and women who have had such childhood experiences often have great joy when they learn how to sing as adults.

I have heard several opera singers describe to me that very difficult but well-written music becomes much more easier to execute when it is included in a dramatic context, which the music is illustrating. This might also speak in favour of the hypothesis that basic aspects of music performing are programmed in us. The speculation is that situations with strong emotional reactions, movements and acts have been automatically associated with basic musical expressions. This would then facilitate learning of the execution of complex pieces of music.

The Finnish neurologist and epidemiologist Hyyppä (2007) has examined possible reasons behind the fact that Swedish-speaking East Bothnians live much longer than Finnish-speaking subjects living in the same region and also longer than Swedish-speaking men and women living in other parts of Finland. His conclusion is that the difference in cardiovascular risk (which is the main component in the difference in longevity) is not due to differences in the prevalence of the "usual" traditional risk factors (smoking, genetic differences, education, physical activity and diet). One has to search for other kinds of risk factors. He claims that a likely explanation of the difference is that the Swedish-speaking East Bothnians have a stronger feeling of cohesiveness than other Finns. Using research terminology, it is claimed that the East Bothnians have a strong "social capital". Choir singing is an important ingredient in this "social capital". It is impossible in the present phase of the development to know how important choir singing may be per se, but the fact that many members in these communities sing in a choir may very well contribute to a feeling of togetherness, not only for those who sing themselves but also for those who listen at gatherings.

Multimodality is an educational principle that has frequently been applied particularly to the education of small children. The basic multimodal principle is that the effect of one modality amplifies the effect of other modalities. Björkvold has discussed this extensively (2005) in relation to the education of children. Children are often training rhythms, rhymes and movements at the same time, and they like very much to do this together with other children. Björkvold argues that rhythm and music are important in education because both modalities and particularly when they are combined can facilitate learning processes, for instance in mathematics and language. There are numerous alphabet song books—easily illustrated by a simple search on Internet. One Swedish example is illustrated in the picture below. This particular alphabet song book (lyrics Lena Anderson, music Kerstin Andeby) uses different species of trees as its common theme. Accordingly, the book uses the two modalities music and text but also stimulates the children's curiosity about nature. The first song is about the ash tree. A free translation is the following: *We have an ash-tree. It's more than hundred years. It's getting taller and taller with years. And I have a see-saw on the lowest bough, where I like to dangle with legs in the air.* This song combines the educational aspirations with a contemporary syncopated musical language (Picture 3.3).

To sing letters facilitates the learning of them. The importance of multimodality is a complication for researchers in the field, however, when they intend to throw light on

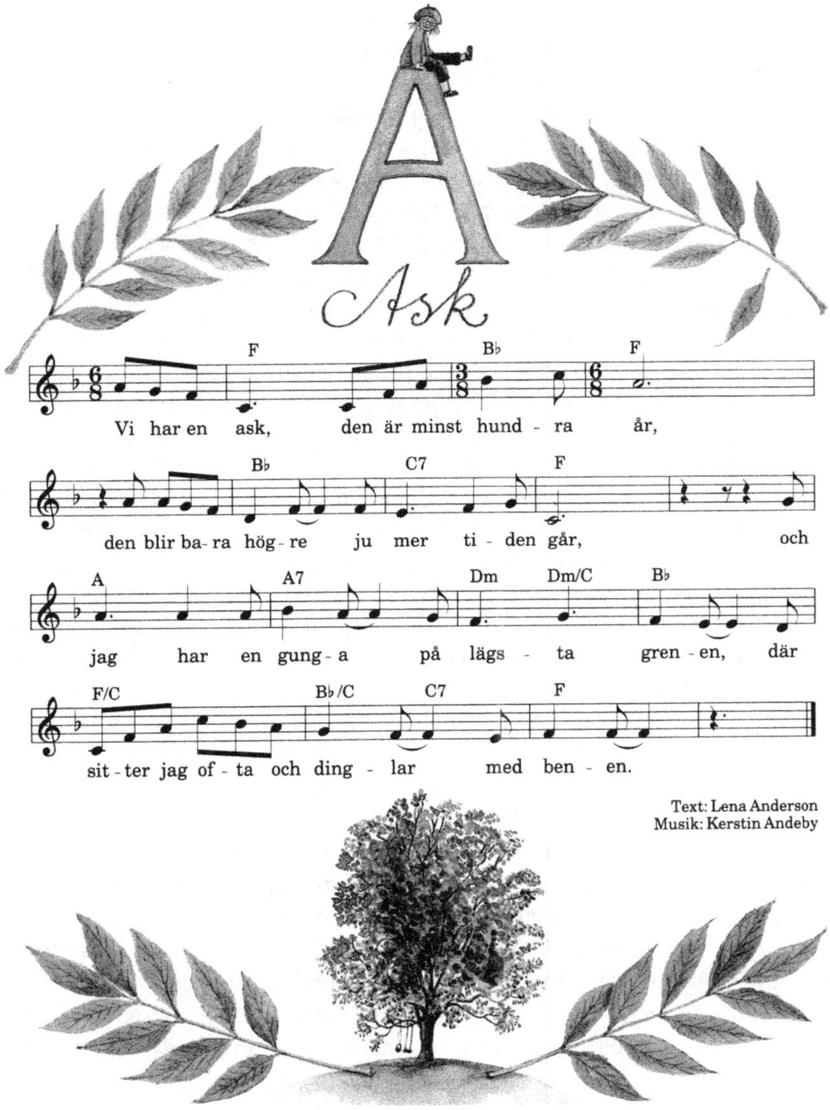
A
Ask
F Bb F
Vi har en ask, den är minst hund - ra år,
Bb C7 F
den blir ba- ra hög- re ju mer ti - den går, och
A A7 Dm Dm/C Bb
jag har en gung - a på lägs - ta gren - en, där
F/C Bb/C C7 F
sit - ter jag of - ta och ding - lar med ben - en.
Text: Lena Anderson
Musik: Kerstin Andeby

Picture 3.3 Ash tree leaves and music notes

the importance of music per se. When music is so intertwined with many other sensory stimuli and these modalities even amplify their effects mutually, it becomes extremely difficult to use accepted scientific methods. One has to understand that the scientific questions may have to be illuminated with other methods than the usual ones.

A British group of researchers (see Burland and Davidson 2004) has performed a series of interviews with people making music, and their focus has been bodily expressions of musical experience. Singers tend to open their hand to the audience when they sing. In the interviews, some music experiences were even giving rise to erotic sensations. This could certainly be comforting—music could replace a lost beloved person. But it may not always be positive! A love partner could also give rise to fatigue, irritation and sadness.

In order to explore the multimodal principle neurobiologically, Baumgartner et al. (2006) performed an interesting experiment on adult persons. They performed functional magnetic resonance brain imaging (filming what goes on in the brain) during three different conditions, during the viewing of a picture in silence, during the listening to a piece of music "intuned with the picture" but without seeing it, and finally when looking at the picture while listening. When the participants looked at the picture during silence, brain areas related to cognitive functions were activated. When they listened to the music without the picture, other areas were activated, all of them related to emotional experiences. During the combined picture/music experience, all of the areas were activated but this activation was stronger than in each one of the other conditions. Accordingly, the combined experience was stronger than the sum of the unimodal experiences. This is a clear demonstration of the ability of music to amplify other kinds of experiences. This may have substantial importance in social contexts, both positively and negatively. To hear music surrounded by a large group of people who send out odours and move and also hear arguments being formulated from a podium is a true multimodal experience. March music accompanying Hitler's talks full of nazi propaganda amplified the hatred against Jews and may have stimulated people to participate in acts that may not have taken place without the music; lowering of the threshold for violence. On the other hand, individuals have also witnessed that they may not have survived difficult circumstances without comforting strong musical experiences. Paul Robertson, a British violinist who is lecturing about the neurological effects of music, has documented the enormous importance that a few well-organised concerts had for the inhabitants of Sarajevo during the siege in the recent Bosnian war.

During the strong social bonding processes that characterise childhood and youth, the musical experience may be particularly important. When I was a student, we gathered singing student songs while we hooked one another's arms rocking together to the rhythm of the music. Perhaps we were then coming close to the ecstatic conditions that are pictured in the cave paintings discussed above. But if we believe that picture, the people in the caves have had much stronger expressions. When today's youth are moving in shadowy light in clubs densely stuffed with people, listening to unbelievably strongly amplified music (unbelievable to the cave people!), they may come closer to the ecstasy of the inhabitants in the caves.

Societal Implications

So far, I have mainly emphasised the positive aspects of music. But there are of course also negative aspects. Music may also make us ill! It is impossible to formulate general principles for health effects of music. Music has a wide diversity, and health can be defined in several ways. Yes, music can also be harmful to health. If we accept that music could be a strong agent for good health, we also have to accept that if we are exposed to the wrong music in the wrong situation when we have had bad experiences of that music previously, it may harm our health. This principle can also be applied to medical drugs. Some life-saving drugs, if prescribed in the wrong dosage and under false premises, may kill. Health effects of a particular piece of music depend upon our previous experiences of the music (which determine what stimulates joy and what stimulates negative emotions), the conditions surrounding us and our own state of mind. Two questions of relevance for society's relationship to music and health could be raised.

I have heard the first question formulated by painters, composers and writers and other professional artists: if we conclude that some kinds of cultural activities improve health, will society demand from the arts that they have to be useful from a health promotion point of view? That could actually be a frightening perspective. An extrapolation would mean that society would not accept cultural activities that have no proved benefit to health. A more general utility perspective is close—how "useful" is a piece of music or a theatre drama? An extreme political application of such thoughts would be the prohibition of "not useful" culture. Hitler's condemnation of *Entartete Musik* ("off the track" music), Stalin's prosecution of artists who produced "anti-Soviet" culture and the Taliban's prohibition of all cultural activities are frightening historical examples. No, music must be allowed to exist on its own premises, and utility demands should not guide cultural policy. But independently of music's demand for freedom of expression, it is beneficial for society that researchers try to systematically describe in what contexts and for whom certain defined kinds of music could improve or harm health.

The second question is about commercialisation of music. There is always a risk, when the power of music is rediscovered, that "not so serious" business wants to earn excessive amounts of money for doing "wonders", for instance curing serious illnesses without scientific evidence. Researchers may be taken hostage in this process, something they have to be aware of. Negative commercialisation is, however, an additional argument for vital research in this area—in order to make society prepared to defend itself.

That music can be used for manipulation is very clear when we consider the use of music in advertisements and commercial movies. When we look at advertisements on television, music is a strong force in influencing our possible decisions. When we buy cinema tickets, we actually pay for being manipulated by the film music. There is a specific "musical grammar" ("semiotics" which the composers of such music are using). This is not revealed to us. Perhaps most of us know intuitively that rapid music with rhythm perceived as faster than one's own heart rate may induce increased heart rate and conversely that a slow rhythm (slower than one's own heart rate) may slow down the pulse. In the same vein, most people would recognise that a strong sound (high sound amplitude) is likely to have a stronger arousal effect than a weak sound. It is probably less well-known that different kinds of chords (disharmonic and harmonic) may have differential psychological and physiological effects—something that will be discussed later in this book. Disharmonic chords mostly (but not always!) correspond to irritated and distressed feelings, whereas harmonic chords correspond to calmer and more agreeable feelings. Whether the melody is moving mainly upwards or downwards, as well as the dominant key (minor or major) are other important dimensions in relation to emotional effects.

We would be able to protect ourselves much more effectively against seductive propaganda if we could increase knowledge about how music influences us. A classical experiment performed by Milliman (1986) showed that customers in a cafeteria were eating more rapidly when music with a fast beat was played than when slow music was played. In a similar vein, people were drinking faster in a bar when fast music was played (McElrea and Standing 1992). Tagg (2006) has discussed the potential importance of increased knowledge among laymen regarding music as a tool for manipulation. Customers would be more able to protect themselves against poorly founded decisions in shops and other similar situations in their daily round of life. Of particular importance is that we would perhaps get a society more able to resist perverse political propaganda. There is a paradox in this, however. As viewers of a film and audience in a concert, we may feel that we do not want to know how we are manipulated! This is a frequent comment that I have heard when I have discussed these matters. It is my impression, however, that knowledge about music manipulation does not take away the intensity and joy of experiencing music! And quite clearly, it would become more difficult to "sell junk" with music manipulation if there would be more general awareness in the population. Tagg (2006) argued that this should be taught to the pupils in schools.

In the next chapter, I will discuss a special case of a social use of music, namely the religious music.

References

Baumgartner, T., Lutz, K., Schmidt, C. F., & Jäncke, L. (2006). The emotional power of music: How music enhances the feeling of affective pictures. *Brain Research, 1075*, 151–164.

Benzon, W. (2001). *Beethoven's Anvil. Music in mind and culture*. New York: Basic Books.

Berg, L. (2005). Gryning över Kalahari. Stockholm: (Dawn over Kalahari) Ordfront.

Björkvold, J.-R. (2005). *Den musiska människan (Musical man)*. Malmö: Runa Förlag.

Brown, S. (2000). Evolutionary models of music: From sexual selection to group selection. In I. Tonneau & N. S. Thompson (Eds.), *Perspective in ethology* (Vol. 13, pp. 231–281)., Evolution, Culture and Behavior New York: Kluwer/Plenum.

Burland, F. K. & Davidson, J. W. (2004). Tracing a musical life transition. Kapitel 4 (sid 225-250) I Davidson JW (redaktör): The Music Practitioner. London : Ashgate.

Clift, S. M. (2012). Singing, wellbeing, and health. In R. Macdonald, G. Kreutz, & L. Mitchell (Eds.), *Music, health & wellbeing* (pp. 113–124). Oxford: Oxford University Press.

De Quadros, A., & Dortewitz, P. (2011). Community, communication, social change: Music in dispossessed Indian communities. *International Journal of Community Music, 4*, 59–70.

Hyyppä, M. T. (2007). *Livskraft ur gemenskap (Life energy from cohesion)*. Lund: Studentlitteratur.

Mc Elrea, H., & Standing, L. (1992). Fast music causes fast drinking. *Perceptual and Motor Skills, 75*, 362.

Milliman, R. E. (1986). The influence of Background music on the behavior of restaurant patrons. *Journal of Consumer Research, 13*, 286–289.

Mithen, S. (2005). *The singing Neanderthals: The origins of music, language, mind and body*. London: Weidenfeld and Nicholson.

Olsson, E. M. G., von Schéele, B., & Theorell, T. (2013). Heart rate variability during choral singing. *Music and Medicine, 5*, 52–59. doi:10.1177/1943862112471399.

Sacks, O. (2007). *Musicophilia. Tales of music and the brain*. London: Picador.

Simkin, R. (1992). Mozart's scatological disorder. *BMJ: British Medical Journal, 305*, 1563–1567.

Tagg, P. (2006). Music, moving images, semiotics and the democratic right to know. In S. Brown & U. Volgsten (Eds.), *Music and manipulation*. New York: Berghahn Books.

Vickhoff, B. (2008). A perspective theory of music perception and emotion. Skrifter från musikvetenskap, Göteborgs universitet, nr 90. ISBN 978 91-85974-06-1, ISSN 1654-6261.

Vickhoff, B., Malmgren, H., Åström, R., Nyberg, G., Engvall, M., Snygg, J., et al. (2013). Music structure determines heart rate variability of singers. *Frontiers in Psychology, 4*, 334. doi:10.3389/fpsyg.2013.00334.

Chapter 4
Music in Religion

Regardless of whether you consider yourself religious or not and of whether you look at yourself as a producer or consumer of music, you are likely to have been exposed to religious music on many occasions. Religious music has a strong tradition going far back in the history of man. That there has been such a large number of music pieces related to religion and that religion has had a high status in society are reasons for the large volume of high-quality religious music. In contrast, the profane music has often had low status. Some of history's most well-known composers and musicians have earned their living from the church, and this has of course contributed to the fact that they have done some of their best pieces for the church. But the religious music also addresses our collectivity, our emotions and our aesthetic experiences. Accordingly, it would be particularly interesting to reflect on religious music when we discuss music and health in general.

For many choir singers, the Mass in B Minor by Johann Sebastian Bach is the favourite piece of all categories. Musically, it has enormous width between weak and "private" to emotionally seeking and intensive and powerful parts. The first movement with the text Kyrie Eleison (Lord, have mercy on us) is special for those of us who are choir tenors—we introduce a lyrical part with a meditative and meandering seeking Kyrie in the high register. From a technical singing point of view, it is a challenge because it has to be quiet and at the same time pregnant. In the last movement Dona nobis pacem (Give us piece), the challenge is different; all the singers have to sing long slow phrases as forcefully as possible without uncontrolled shouting.

What makes some of the church music so moving? The religious music is the basis for a substantial part of all the music that is performed in the world. This is true even in countries where religion does not have a strong position—as in Northern Europe. Many choir singers go to their rehearsals in the church despite the fact that they do not look at themselves as believers. I belong to that category myself. I went to the rehearsals even during the late 1960s and early 1970s when many of us were strongly critical of society (including the state church) and disliked church rituals and practice. To be a choir singer at a church actually also included participation in church services, not only in concerts.

T. Theorell, *Psychological Health Effects of Musical Experiences*,
SpringerBriefs in Psychology, DOI: 10.1007/978-94-017-8920-2_4,

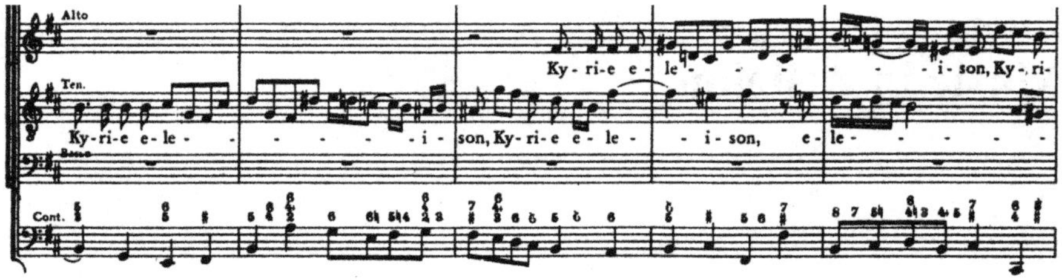

The religious music has probably existed throughout man's history. Today, it is impossible to hear the music that was played in Egypt 3,000 years ago, but there are pictures showing that it existed. And similar pictures exist from other ancient cultures, for instance the Maya culture.

In our own church in our time, we are affected by the religious contents and the moments of meditation in the music. Often, the words are in Latin which means that the emotional effects of the words themselves are small since most of us simply do not understand Latin. And even when we understand the words, they may not engage us so much. For instance, "*Oh God's Lamb you take away the sins of the world*" may not be an effective message since we do not sacrifice lambs nowadays—although we know that the text should be interpreted symbolically. Strong effects are therefore often caused almost entirely by the music and its framework.

In the passions of Bach, we are also participating in a dramatic sequence of events. We are staging events that have a strong existential meaning for all human beings—Jesus suffering and dying as well as the scorning and torturing of him. For a northern European, the language, German, is more easy to understand than Latin. Of course, the words in such a drama affect us deeply.

The physical characteristics of the musical church space are often impressive. High ceiling and long reverberation of sound. The music has a stronger impact in such a room than in a small room with "dry" acoustics. This contributes to the strong emotional power of the church music (Wilson Dickson 1992).

That the religious music has very old traditions has been extensively documented. In the bible, the early references to music are only indirect, but for instance in Miriam's song in the second book of Moses, there is a very concrete reference to music performance:

And the lady prophet Miriam, Aron's sister, grasped a kettle drum, and all the women accompanied her with kettle drums and dancing. And Miriam sang to them...

Wilson-Dickson has summarised the power of the religious music in the following dimensions:

1. The extatic dimension. This corresponds among other things to the biological upbeat (arousal) effect of a high tempo and the downbeat (deceleration) effect of a low tempo. The physical aspects—such as vibrations in the room—may be of considerable importance.
2. The symbolic dimension. During the second century AC Clemens from Alexandria wrote: (God's creation song) gave rise to a consonant universe and he even tuned the dissonance of the elements to consonant chords in order to

make the whole cosmos harmonic. According to Wilson-Dickson: "*In this way the music that was composed and played by human beings became a symbol of the eternally larger patterns and coincidences that existed in God's creation*". This can be perceived strongly in the B Minor Mass, for instance in the Credo movement.
3. The affect dimension. The main task of the music is to communicate feelings. A melody constitutes to many people (for instance to me) a much more powerful means of expressing feelings than speech.

These three dimensions are of course not isolated from one another. Sometimes, they exist jointly, which is the case with the passion music during Easter. With regard to the affect dimension, in these monumental pieces of music, there are wide swings between the aggressiveness and arousal in the demands from the Hebrews that Jesus should die to our sadness that he has died and the celebration of his resurrection. There are oscillations between physical effects of violent crescendos of almost painful loudness and vibrations to whispering quiet parts. Of course, there is a strong extatic component in all of this as well. The symbolic dimension is to a great part the comforting function. We may feel comfort because we feel that we are included in something much bigger than ourselves. One does not have to be religious to experience comfort in the thought that we are part of nature's life and death cycle. All of this is mediated by the acoustic experiences in the church room.

Finally, the music amplifies the feelings embedded in the moment. When we listen to funeral services, this is often because someone close has recently died. Parts of the requiem music by Mozart (Lacrimosa), for instance, are often used at funerals, and these pieces help the listeners to focus on their sadness. Listeners often know that Mozart himself was dying when he composed this music, and this certainly influences the listening. It may be that the music that has the strongest influence on us is often composed by a composer who experienced strong sadness or joy when he or she wrote it. Johann Sebastian Bach was influenced by his mother's spiritism. After his first wife had died unexpectedly when he was away travelling, he composed his partitas for solo violin. These are filled with coded religious messages. Among many things, each one of the tone numbers in the scale corresponds to a number in the alphabet. In this way, Bach was able to write religious messages to us. Most listeners do not have the faintest idea about this, but it is likely that there is some influence, at least since the intensity of the music may become stronger while this is ongoing.

The religious music has been strongly circumvented by strict rules. There are examples of composers who have been banned by the church when they crossed borders. The strict rules may have created a feeling of security in the church rituals. At the same time, however, even small surprises produce strong effects when the rules are so strict. In Fauré's requiem, there is one movement, Pie Jesu, who is frequently sung by a boy soprano. The subtle changes in key in this piece create surprises causing tension in the midst of all the calmness that dominates the piece. Not surprisingly, Fauré wrote this music in a sad period—after his father's premature death.

Despite the strict rules for the religious music, the border between religious and profane music is not always as clear as we might believe. Verdi's requiem could be regarded as a church opera, and Mozart's requiem also has operatic elements. Already Claudio Monteverdi who lived between 1567 and 1643 composed both opera and church music, and sometimes, it is clear that his church oratorios have borrowed traits from the opera. The most well-known of Monteverdi's church oratorios is Vesper della Beata Vergine which may have been originally a collection of compositions made for very different occasions and purposes. Some of the texts in the Vesper tell us about the erotically flavoured admiration of Virgin Maria that was common at the time. Texts from the Songs in the bible were allowed despite the fact that these texts are love declarations with physical expressions.

Gospel choirs represent a tradition with unusually strong cohesiveness. Gospel choirs have been strong institutions in the USA. In the gospel choir, men and women who have been living under strong oppression have had an outlet for strong emotions. The cohesiveness has released energy that enables the participants to make fantastic musical performances. In such performances, both the extatic and the emotional dimension are represented. The strong cohesiveness corresponds to the symbolic dimension. I have witnessed services with gospel singing, one in Harlem in New York and one in Texas. Choir plays a powerful role as mediator of emotions and amplifier of cohesiveness. Although I was a passive audience, I was strongly affected by the powerful emotions. Many participants in gospel singing are surprised by the singing resources they have. In the extatic state that they experience, they are suddenly able to perform very advanced singing. This may speak in favour of the idea that there is more of music performing ability programmed in us and that this may be evident when inhibitions go away. From Americans, I have also heard the comment—from people who do not regard themselves as musical and not particularly religious—that they go to church because they want to sing together with others. A good illustration of the association between religion and music.

In the next chapter, we shall discuss more in detail what happens when one listens to music.

Reference

Wilson-Dickson, A. (1992). *The story of Christian music*. Oxford: Lion Publishers.

Chapter 5
Music for Body and Soul: Physiological Effects of Listening to Music

Music starts processes in the brain, which in turn affect the whole body. What do we know more in detail about these? Here, I shall examine what neurobiological research tells us and what this knowledge could possibly teach us about the musical experience (Fig. 5.1).

The American neurobiologist Joseph Le Doux (1998) made the discovery with his co-workers some years ago that emotionally charged sound stimuli are transmitted in the brain via two different routes, which he labelled the "upper" and the "lower". The same routes could also be labelled the "slower" and the "faster" route. The sound impulse first reaches a relay station in the thalamus located in the midbrain. A musical tune may be associated with anxiety. If this is the case, the faster lower route transmits the impulse to the amygdala, which has an important role in stress and anxiety reactions. The amygdala, which is part of the emotional brain, rapidly triggers a stress response in the brain and the rest of the body. The emotional brain is a primitive part of our brain, which can also be found in most animals.

The impulse is also transmitted via the higher route up to the brain cortex, which processes the cognitive interpretation. (Which piece? Where did I hear this before? Does it mean danger?) If the cognitive analysis leads to the conclusion that the situation associated with the music is dangerous, an impulse is sent to the amygdala from the cortex as well. Since this transmittal is much slower, the amygdala has already reacted, but the cortex reaction can now modify the primitive stress reaction. If the sound impulse lasts for a very short moment (for instance a dissonant chord disappearing rapidly), the cognitive cortex may never become aware of the phenomenon and may therefore not be able to process the information. In such a case, it is only the lower route that has been activated, and the brain may never become aware of the source of the anxiety reaction. This has been clearly shown in brain research on picture perception. If simplified pictures of neutral, sad, happy and angry faces are shown in random order very rapidly, the person will not be able to know cognitively which faces he or she has seen. But functional magnetic brain imaging (a method for studying activation of different

T. Theorell, *Psychological Health Effects of Musical Experiences*, SpringerBriefs in Psychology, DOI: 10.1007/978-94-017-8920-2_5,

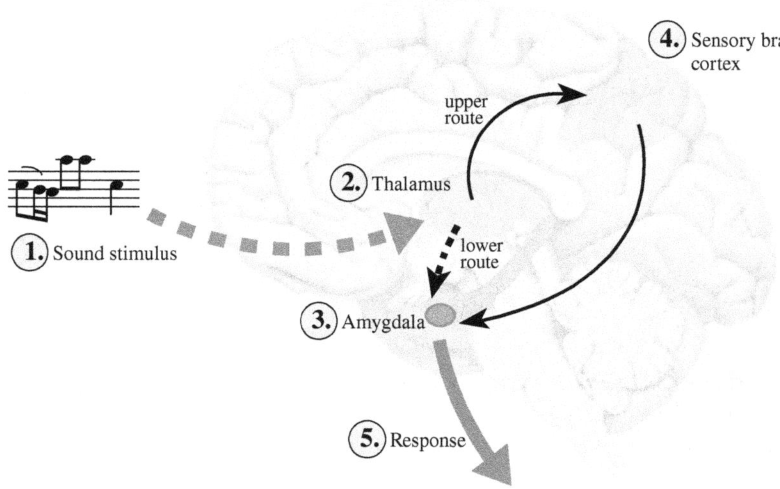

Fig. 5.1 The emotional brain. Sound impulses are transmitted along two different routes when they reach the brain. Via the lower (and *faster*) route, incomplete emotional information reaches the amygdala (and other parts of the emotional brain) while the complete information reaches the emotional brain much later after having been transmitted via the upper (and *slower*) route to the cognitive brain and then to the emotional brain. *Source* Le Doux. ©Annika Röhl, Töres Theorell

parts of the brain during simulation) shows that the amygdala is activated every time the angry face is shown but not when the other faces are shown—despite the fact that the person cannot say when it is the angry face that turns up.

Is there any specific part of the brain that corresponds to musical experiences? No, it is not that simple. But there are regions in the brain that are activated and which collaborate when musical processes are ongoing. And when certain parts of the brain are injured, our ability to experience music may be affected. The parts that are important for musical experiences are partly overlapping with those processing speech, for instance. There is one region in the brain, the planum temporale in the left hemisphere, that is associated with absolute pitch, the ability to know exactly which tone is played or sung. The person with absolute pitch will know when I play an A and correspondingly, if I ask that person to sing an A he/she will immediately be able to do so without hesitating. This unusual ability is more common among musicians than in others, but it is not per se associated with the ability to perform music well (Fagius 2002).

The situation surrounding a music experience is of great importance. For instance if a musical piece is being played after a person has been instructed to tell which piece it is and what chords it contains, it is mainly the left hemisphere that is activated. On the other hand, if the person is asked to tell whether the chord is false or not, it is mainly the right hemisphere that is activated. Both hemispheres are important but in different ways, the left one has more to do with cognition while the right side is more important to integrated "total" interpretation. There is considerable scientific support for the notion that the spontaneous "total" musical experience in a non-professional listener mainly activates the right half of the brain. The more professional the listener is, the more activation of the left hemisphere, so in the professional brain both the right and the left hemispheres are activated.

Another way of saying this is that professional music education transforms the musical experience increasingly into a cognitive one. The more I have been taught about music, the more I wonder which piece is being played, which tempo, why certain intensity was chosen etc. The more "naive" we are, we perceive the music in a more holistic way corresponding only to a "right brain" activation.

That people are strongly affected by music has been noticed by many. The music psychology professor Alf Gabrielsson (2011) recruited more than 900 subjects for an interesting study. He asked people to describe in their own words the most profound musical experience that they had had in their lives. He also tried to categorise these experiences with regard to contents, context, consequences etc. Gabrielsson stated that it is very difficult to do such a categorisation since the experiences cover a very large area. Music seems to comprise the "whole psychological reality". Many of these situations have meant turning points in the subjects' lives. There are examples of subjects in deep depression who "discovered" a kind of music that they had never been interested in before but in this situation they became passionately engaged in listening to this kind of music, which helped them out of the depression. The enormous variation of themes in these stories may not be so surprising in view of the fact that music could amplify the emotional state that we happen to be in for the moment. Music can act both as a stimulating and as a relaxing agent. There is extensive published research showing that the body is reacting that way when one listens to music. Music which is "right" (right for the person and the situation) can "vitalise". This could correspond to increased heart rate and concentration of stress hormones (such as cortisol). It can also activate secretion of the body's own morphine (endorphins), raise blood pressure, increase the tendency for the body to form clots (coagulation) and furthermore increase the activity in some parts of the immune system (for instance immune globulins). And, as I just pointed out, the reversed pattern has been observed when relaxing music is being played, lowered heart rate, lowered blood pressure etc.

One of the studies of physiological effects of music listening showed that the concentration of cortisol (a hormone with an important role in the mobilisation of energy in stressful situations) in saliva (Khalfa et al. 2003) decreased much more rapidly after a standardised stress situation in the laboratory when the subjects listened to suitable music than when they did not listen. A valuable review of psychophysiological effects (heart rate, blood pressure, constriction of blood vessels in the periphery and sweating) of music listening in relation to stressful experiences was published already many years ago by Barlett (1996).

Composers have always applied practical knowledge regarding emotional effects of different types of music. Mozart's operas and modern musicals have this in common, the composer manipulates our feelings. The same could be said about film music and music in advertisements. When we go to the cinema, we even pay to be manipulated by the music! Some basic characteristics seem to have predictable effects on the majority of people in the audience. For instance a tempo that is higher than our heart rate, strong volume and high pitch are factors usually associated with arousal. A tempo lower than our heart rate, low volume and low pitch are correspondingly associated with the opposite physiological changes. The characteristics of chords are also important since harmonic chords may contribute to calmness and disharmonic ones to anxiety. However, the effect of chords could vary in different cultures since what is perceived as harmonic differs in different traditions. The individual's previous experiences also make a difference. I myself may during some circumstances feel relaxed when I listen to music with many disharmonic chords. This is probably because my own musical experiences sometimes make me relate these kinds of chords to relaxed conditions. Music dominated by upward movements may be vitalizing, whereas slow movements downwards could amplify feelings of fear. Combinations of all these characteristics give rise to very complex effects. A team of researchers (Krumhansl et al. 1997) have described how a group of individuals reacted physiologically to three different kinds of musical pieces which were assumed to induce *sadness* (Albinoni: "Adagio" and Barber: "Adagio"), *fear* (Mussorgski: "Witch hill", Holt: "March" in "Planets") and *joy* (Vivaldi: "Spring" in "The Seasons" and Alfvén: "Midsummer wake"), respectively. First of all, it was shown that the music really induced the expected feelings in most experimental subjects. Secondly, it turned out that the physiological reactions were indeed different in these induced emotional states. During the sad music, the persons had lower heart rate, higher blood pressure and more sweating (galvanic skin response). When the fearful music was played, there was an increased respiratory rate (number of breaths per minute) and decreased blood flow in the periphery (finger tips). The joyful music was associated mainly with an increased respiratory rate.

Many have experienced chills while listening to music. According to Panksepp (1995) who has examined this systematically, music associated with sadness and melancholy is the most common kind of music that could trigger the strong reaction due to a contraction of the small muscles at the root of the hair sacs in the skin, for instance on the arms. These small muscles are influenced by the autonomic nervous system so it is not so surprising that these kinds of reactions might arise. Why we have this reaction is unknown. The explanation may be found in the evolution from animal to man. For instance it could be that an animal that expands the volume of the fur in a sad situation looks bigger and more impressive, something that may have been of importance in threatening sad situations? It could also be that expansion of the fur volume could have been important as a protection against cold temperatures which could be a problem in a situation when the animal is hiding and is not allowed to move? Blood and Zatorre (2001) performed a thorough examination of five male and five female students at a music conservatory in Canada. They selected a piece that they knew would give rise to chills. When this particular piece was being played, they exhibited a strong increase in heart rate, electrical activity in muscles and increased breathing depth. The physiological changes were more pronounced when they listened to this piece than when they listened to other kinds of music. With PET scanning (positron emission tomography), a method that is used for the study of changes in blood flow in different parts of the brain, it was shown that during the thrills these persons had an increased blood flow in those parts of the brain that are associated with reward and agreeable feelings. The researchers doing this study discussed their finding and speculated that there are parallels between this reaction and the reactions that arise in the brain during sexual experiences and during eating good food. They also make the parallel with drug addiction. A more recently published study of one person who unexpectedly reacted with chills listening to improvised piano music—when the improvisation went from calming and harmonic sequences to more irregular rhythm and disharmonic chords (Vickhoff et al. 2012). It so happened that several physiological functions were recorded "online" in the subject while this happened. The recordings showed that the physiological reactions to the change in the music started with a slight increase in heart rate as well as diminished variation in heart rate. After this, sweating (recorded in the finger) increased. Finally, the finger skin temperature started to decrease. Within 40 s, a 0.7° C decrease in skin temperature was observed.

To weep is also a common reaction while listening to sad music. Weeping also has a phylogenetic meaning: few affective expressions are as effective in making surrounding people offer help and support! But the circumstances are also important. If I am irritated and aroused, I could become even more irritated if somebody plays quiet and soft music. To conclude, music is a powerful tool but bodily effects are sometimes hard to predict. One example from our own research may serve as an illustration. The diversified psychophysiological reaction patterns during listening to various kinds of music have been described from laboratory experiments by Krumhansl and collaborators (1997).

My student, Joseph Lingham, had other students and employees at the Karolinska Institute select two of their own favourite music pieces. One of them should be stimulating, and the other one relaxing according to what the participants thought themselves. Having made their choices, they were placed comfortably in a chair with a listening device. Psychophysiological equipment was applied so that among other things heart rate and breathing frequency could be recorded. They first sat quietly without music and then a random half of them listened to the stimulating piece. Then, silence again and subsequently the relaxing piece. The other randomised half of the participants started with the relaxing piece—we did not want the order in which the pieces were being played to have any influence on the findings. Movements were not allowed during the experiment. Figure 5.2 shows how different the changes in heart rate were in the 37 individuals. Two of them had a very pronounced increase in heart rate from silence, 20 beats per minute, when they listened to the stimulating music. One of these two participants also had a very pronounced lowering of heart rate, 20 beats per minute, during listening to the music that she thought would be relaxing. Accordingly, there was a difference between the two listening experiences in this individual of 40 beats per minute.

On the whole, the stimulating music was associated with a clear and statistically significant acceleration of heart rate. The average increase was seven beats per minute compared with the quiet condition when the heart rate was between

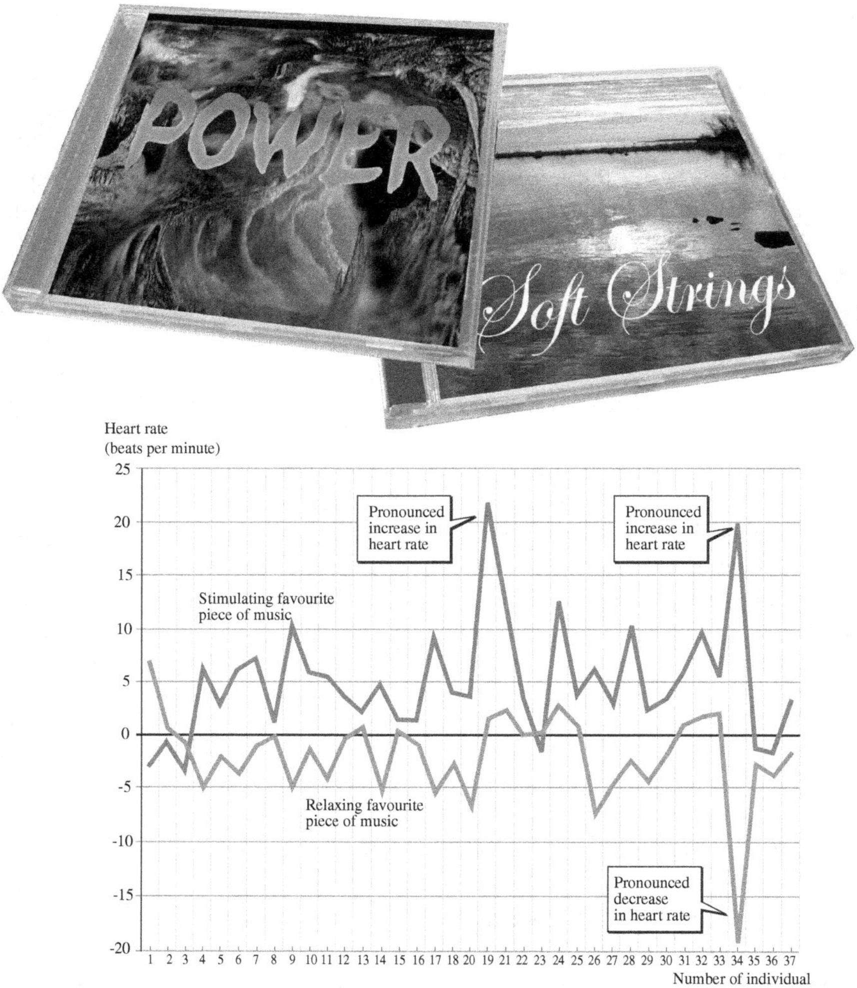

Fig. 5.2 Emotional effect. The diagram shows heart rate change from silence to music in 37 individuals. The heart rate showed a pronounced increase when the persons listened to favourite music (*red*) that they had selected as "stimulating". The effect tended to be in the opposite direction—albeit less consistent—when they listened to favourite music (*blue*) that they had selected as "relaxing". In one individual, the difference between the extremes was 40 beats per minute. ©Annika Röhl

50 and 70 beats per minute. The "relaxing" music, on the other hand, did not produce the expected deceleration of heart rate in some individuals. Quite to the contrary, in eleven cases, it was even associated with an increased heart rate. There were similar observations with regard to breathing. During the stimulating music, the breathing frequency increased significantly and the average increase was four breathing cycles per minute. During "relaxing" music, there was no significant change. Emotional self-recordings verified this in the psychological

domain, whereas the stimulating music quite clearly induced arousal feelings, the "relaxing" piece triggered both relaxed and aroused feelings. The conclusion to be drawn from this seems to be that these highly educated people were skilful in selecting their own stimulating music, but they were not as successful with regard to "relaxing" music—it frequently did not have the expected calming effect on heart rate and breathing. If breathing increases without proportion to physical needs, a number of physical symptoms may arise. Most people know that hyperventilation may induce fainting. In the corresponding way, a strong stimulating music effect may induce vertigo due to a lowered carbon dioxide content in the blood. Such strong effects may even induce constriction of some of the brain arteries—amplifying this effect.

Perhaps this small experiment (Lingham and Theorell 2009) may illustrate music's role in modern society. While the most commonly stated belief regarding music and health is that music is relaxing, most of our listening to music seems to be for stimulation and vitalisation. And music is frequently used in order to increase the arousal level even when this is not health promoting. For instance many adolescents use music for staying awake at night when they should be sleeping.

There are differences in reactions to one and the same piece of music that are not due to previous musical experiences. For instance it has been shown that self-reported personality patterns may make a difference. Such differences become clear when students describe individual attitudes to background music when they study. Daoussis and Mc Kelvie (1986) showed that students who described themselves as extroverts frequently listened to music when studying (50 %) while introverts did much less frequently (25 %). In both groups, they pointed out that the volume was low when they used music in this way and also that wordless music was more acceptable than songs with words—which could distract.

As I pointed out, the Lingham experiment may illustrate that in our time men and women are more able to select stimulating than relaxing music. This may be an important reason why no physiological evidence of relaxation was recorded in several cases. Two participants who had an increased heart rate while listening to "relaxing" music had selected love songs, which may in fact be clearly arousing for many people. Perhaps today's emphasis on the importance of a high tempo could partly explain this. So maybe many subjects in the general population lack the skill of identifying relaxing agents in their lives. It has been proven in many scientific studies that pieces of music selected for relaxation by experts (music therapists), collaborating with the participants themselves do induce a decreased psychophysiological arousal level. Some hundred years ago, this knowledge may have been more widespread. It may not be a coincidence that there are parallels between activity in structures related to rhythm in the brain and rhythmic structures in some types of oriental music. Bettermann and others (2002) have formulated the hypothesis that rhythmic structures in music may have been invented because human beings have had a bodily perception of their own biological rhythms related to cardiovascular and respiratory function. Bernardi and Sleight (2007) have shown that the monotonous recital of many catholic prayers has a pace that the respiration and cardiac functions try to synchronise with.

Bernardi and Sleight have furthermore shown that the monotonous repetition of Catholic prayers or yoga manthras are synchronising breathing with parts of heart rate variability (low frequency power). This part of heart rate variability is related to the activity in the sympathetic nervous system, and one result of the synchronisation could be that the sympathetic nervous system is lowering its activity while the parasympathetic counter regulatory system is activated when these prayers or manthras are being read. Similar observations have been made for slow hymns in folk songs, for instance traditional ones from Dalecarlia in Sweden.

Also, when you listen to music, there is an adaptation of heart rate and breathing to the rhythm and character of the music. One study by Bernardi et al. showed a very clear relationship between rhythm and breathing frequency and in that experiment other aspects of the music were unimportant. Two types of slow music (raga and slow classical music) corresponded to approximately the same breathing frequency (around 15 breaths per minute), while rap, techno music and classical music with a higher tempo corresponded to considerably higher breathing frequency (17–18 breaths per minute). There are however also specific effects of different types of music and research on this subject has been very detailed.

In the research performed by Krantz et al. (2006), it has been shown that lay people (non-musicians) in Sweden react in a predictable way when diatonic ascending chords (two notes at the same time) are being played. Minor second (two notes as close as possible to one another on a twelve tone scale, for instance c and c sharp) and major seventh (two notes that are as almost and as close as possible to an octave, for instance A and a flat) are the most disharmonic diatonic chords. When these chords are being played, the experimental persons tend to report disharmonic emotions, such as worry, irritation and sadness. Chords in the middle range tend to trigger soft or agreeable feelings. Examples are minor third (for instance the sound of most cuckoos), major third (for instance the famous start in Beethoven's fifth symphony), fourth (for instance the start of Lohengrin's first aria in Wagner's opera—"In fernem Land…") and fifth (for instance the start of "Twinkle little star" or "Ba ba little Sheep"). One additional example is the major sixth that is mostly associated with exuberant joy (for instance the first interval in Tamino's aria ("Magic Flute" by Mozart) when he sees the image of Tamina and immediately falls in love with it. In Krantz' research on spontaneous bodily movements corresponding to the different chords, the major sixth was associated with the most pronounced joy whereas a sensation of wholeness was the most strongly associated with the fifth.

These kinds of observations could be taken one step further. By means of continuous recordings of electrocardiograms, we recorded the heart rate variability in subjects who listened randomly to either major third or major seventh (Krantz et al. 2010). These were non-professionals so they should be regarded as average people. When they were not allowed to move, there was a clear difference between the two situations. Heart rate showed much less variation when the subjects listened to the major third than when they listened to the major seventh. My interpretation of this may be speculative; there is a disagreeable "scary" element in the surprise effect when the major seventh is played. This may trigger an exaggerated parasympathetic "disgust" reaction. The experiment further showed that there was less effect of the major seventh when it was being played the second time and that the difference between the cardiovascular effects of the two intervals disappeared when the subjects were allowed to move freely in the room. The major third on the other hand may have "calmed the heart". It should be pointed out that the most frequently utilised measure, number of heart beats per minute, did not differ in the two situations. Accordingly, it was necessary to do a more detailed analysis, patterns of variations in heart rate, to discover this reaction. When music is used in torture, the use of disharmonic chords is frequent. In the torture situation, the victim is often prevented from moving; he or she may be tied to a chair. Our own experiment was very far from torture, but it may be of interest that the combination of restricted movement and a disharmonic chord had a particularly powerful disturbing effect on the heart.

A more detailed and scholarly discussion of the complex relationships between music and emotion can be found in Juslin and Sloboda (2013). See also Boso et al. (2006).

That heart and lungs synchronise with music may not be surprising to the reader. More surprising is that there may also be musical experiences mirrored in other sensory reactions that we may not think of. The professional word for this is synaesthesia. I have heard from many musicians that different "keys" (for instance A minor or D major) correspond to different colours. Another example is the association with gustatory sensations. Beeli et al. (2005) described a musician who associated different music intervals with different tastes, minor second with sour, major second with bitter, minor third with salt, major third with sweet etc. Minor seventh corresponded to bitter and major seventh to sweet. Accordingly, the tastes in the two ends of the octave were the same. We could also take music reactions to unexpected bodily domains. New research tools make it possible for us to record what goes on in most parts of the body while subjects listen to music. For instance there could also be a direct effect on the movements in the gastrointestinal system. In one experiment (Chen et al. 2005), an equipment recording pressure changes was introduced into the ventricle. It was shown that sound influenced the patterns of pressure changes. Calm music induced slow coordinated movements (bradygastria), while disorganised noise was associated with fibrillating rapid uncoordinated movements. It is well known in psychosomatic medicine that the gut and the ventricle are sensitive organs that react to all kinds of psychological stressors. Biochemical bodily processes are also influenced when you listen to music. One example is the secretion of immunoglobulin A in saliva, which is influenced by musical experiences (Rider et al. 1990). Maybe this could have significance for the resistance to infections. In many activities typical to the modern world, music is used in ways that may seem "new" but are in fact very old. A striking example is the music that is played in the gym. Special kinds of music have been developed for this. One is reminded of the music that has been used in the history of man in order to facilitate physical work, for instance "pulling boat songs", sailor songs for rowing or managing big sails and march music for facilitating long troop walks. I had my own experiences of march music during my military service (which was compulsory in Sweden when I was a young man). I almost felt like flying when march music was played during marches. Neurologists have pointed out that the patellar (knee) reflex is amplified when march music is being played, so it has been known for a long time that music influences neurological functions.

A modern line of research has shown that specially adapted music may decrease both the subjective experience of physical effort and the physiological reactions to it. Szmedra and Bacharach (1998) for instance did such an experiment about 10 years ago. Young men were asked to do exactly the same physical work on the treadmill during two different conditions. One was to run in silence, and the other was while listening to special gym music. The two conditions were randomly ordered. The blood concentration of lactic acid was assessed. Heart rate and blood pressure were recorded, and the subjects were asked to make a self-rating of effort. Despite the fact that the physical work was fixed and exactly the same in the two parts of the experiment, blood pressure and heart rate elevation were smaller during the music condition and the same observation was made for subjective effort and lactic acid concentration. Other researchers have made similar observations. So how is it possible that one and the same amount of physical work can be made with less biological cost with "gym music" than without it? One explanation could be that the physical movements may be more efficiently coordinated with music—resulting in more efficient biology. Another explanation could be that hormonal effects contribute to improved energy use, for instance by improved distribution of blood to muscles.

Other research in this field has shown that in long-distance cycling (10 km), when the cyclists choose their own tempo, listening to fast dance music ("trance" with tempo 142 beats per minute) is likely to induce an elevated cycling tempo and the work being perceived as harder than without music (Atkinson et al. 2004). In another study, the effects of different types of music on heart rate, rating of perceived exertion and time to exhaustion were studied. The subjects performed their physical work on a treadmill, and the conditions were randomly allocated to "soft music", "loud, fast and exciting music" and silence. The results showed that the soft music reduced physiological and psychological arousal during submaximal exercise and also increased endurance of performance (Copeland and Franks 1991)

The real challenge for research today is to answer the following question: can regularly repeated listening to (or performing) music promote health by stimulating good forces in the body? Some minor studies have been related to the most recent ideas in biological science. They have examined whether music experiences could favourably influence the interplay between genes and environment in health promotion.

As outlined above, the definition of the stress concept that I have chosen is "the arousal that occurs when energy is needed in a demanding or challenging situation". This arousal is not dangerous in itself—it is necessary in many situations and could even save lives. But when it becomes long lasting and is not interrupted by recuperation and relaxation the body may be hurt. High levels of stress hormones lasting for long periods could be dangerous in their own right but equally important is that the ability of the body to repair and restore worn out cells is hampered by long-lasting stress periods. The interplay between genes and environment is envisaged by the assumption that dangerous genes could be "sleeping", non-activated, as long as the environment is calm. However, if the body is repeatedly exposed to markedly demanding or challenging situations those genes become activated and then they may give rise to a number of bodily reactions. Among many things, there may be reactions in the immune system, indicating that the body is constantly aroused. Bittman et al. (2005) performed a study of health care employees. Genes related to the stress reactions in the immune system were examined before and after a music and dance programme had been instituted as well as in a control group. The programme *Recreational Music Making* (RMM) contained rhythmic exercises with drums and dancing movements once a week. There was evidence when the intervention group was compared with the control group that RMM may have "deactivated" the studied stress genes—that these did not respond as vividly to stress agents as they did before the programme. Such changes were not seen in the control group. This was a small study that may be criticised methodologically, and it should therefore be regarded as a pilot study. However, the basic idea is very interesting. The same group of researchers has also been able to show that this programme (RMM) may reduce the risk of developing the "burnout syndrome" among student nurses (Bittman et al. 2004)

The ability of the body to regenerate worn out cells has been less extensively studied in relation to musical experiences, but some results are described in the chapter on choir music in this book.

Passive and Active

A question that is frequently posed when possible health promoting effects of musical experiences are discussed is whether passive regular consumption of music may have as strong effects on health as active regularly occurring performance of music. This question has not been examined in so many studies. The professor of social medicine Lars Olof Bygren with colleagues (Bygren et al. 1996) found in their prospective cohort studies of randomly selected Swedes that men and women who had "consumed culture" at least once a week had increased longevity and better health than other Swedes. This finding was true even after possible confounders such as health at start, socio-economic conditions and health-related life style factors (such as smoking habits) had been taken into account. Väänänen et al. (2009) have reported similar findings from an even larger population study in Finland. There are many methodological difficulties to be solved in this kind of research, however. Bygren and his group of researchers (2009) have prolonged their study and made it more sophisticated. These later studies seem to show that frequent participation in cultural activities protects mainly against the development of cancer. The researchers speculated that this could be due to possible favourable effects of culture consumption on parts of the immune system that are important for the body's defence against cancer development.

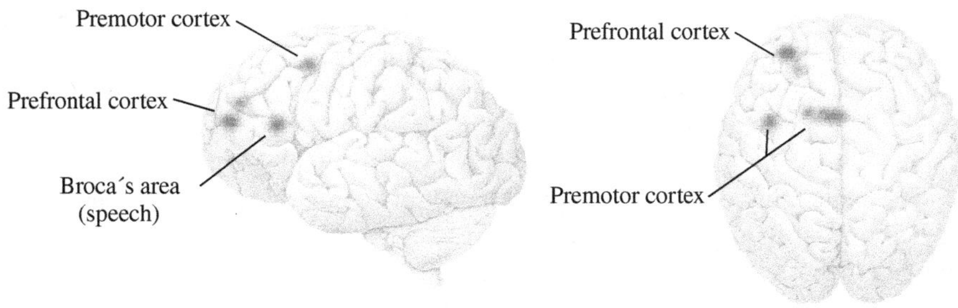

Fig. 5.3 Passive listening to rhythms activates the brain's motor regions. The picture shows brain regions that are activated when experimental subjects were listening to a stable pulse without making movements. Several motor regions, those activating muscle movements and those influencing speech, were activated. A possible explanation is that in these regions mirror neurons that are active when we are producing rhythms are also activated when we listen to rhythms. The picture is modified from Sara L Bengtsson et al. (2009) Cortex 45:62–79

In these latter publications, however, there is no evidence that actively performing music would be more health promoting than simply "consuming" music (defined as attending concerts) at least once week. The borderline between "active" and "passive" may not be so clear cut as many readers may believe. Every cultural experience has a social connotation. If I am watching a movie on television at home, it is likely that I am going to discuss the contents of this movie with others and then even this very passive consumption has a social effect. Those who are actively performing music will also have many more passive experiences than others. The person playing or singing may not play or sing all the time. During long periods, he or she listens while others are playing or singing.

That increased participation in cultural activities can have profound effects in elderly was shown in a controlled real-life experiment many years ago. Elderly subjects in one experimental ward were followed through a period of 6 months when they were grouped with other elderly according to their own hobby (cultural) interests. Group activities based upon these hobbies were facilitated by the staff. Improvements with regard to physiological, social and psychological parameters were observed during the study period in the active group, whereas no such effects were observed in the control ward (Arnetz et al. 1983) (Fig. 5.3).

"Mirror neurons" is, as we have seen, a concept which corresponds to the fact that a person looking at somebody doing something concomitantly activates the cells in his/her brain that correspond exactly to that act. If there is a movement performed by the active person's hands, the brain cells corresponding to those hand movements are activated in the passive person in the same way as they are activated in the active person. This does not pertain only to movements (motor neurons) but is also applicable to emotions and is the basis of human empathy. The existence of such processes may explain part of the power of music (Vickhoff 2008). It also wipes out absolute borders between "passive" and "active" musical experiences. In order to make the mirror neurons work, it is necessary for the listener to have heard the piece before. He or she should also be able, at least to some extent, to perform the particular piece (for instance vocalise it). It may be the combination of predictability, which means that we are "making" the music in our heads and even are one step ahead of it, and unexpected developments in it that constitute interesting musical experiences. All of a sudden the musician/singer makes a new loop that we can accept in the circumstances. The really interesting music is constructed exactly in that way, with a combination of predictability and surprise. This may be applicable to any kind of music.

In research that our group made in Västernorrland (a county in northern Sweden), the immediate emotional reactions to different kinds of cultural "passive" activities in employees in four different work sites were recorded. Different types of cultural performances were offered, these selected employees once a week for 3 months (Hartzell and Theorell 2007). The producers of these performances were regional theatre groups, music bands/orchestras, dance troups etc. A wide range of experiences was offered, such as chamber music, pop music, jazz, theatre and movie. The emotional experiences were assessed by means of simple and direct measures, so-called visual analogue scales. There was one scale for vitality (ranging from extreme tiredness to the left to extreme vitality to the right) and one other for joy (from extreme sadness to the left to extreme joy to the right). Participants were asked to rate vitality and joy on the horizontal scale before every cultural event started and immediately after it. The difference between the "after" and the "before" assessment was calculated for every event and every person. A clear pattern that we saw was that the "vitality effect" (increase from before to after) of the cultural event was stronger whenever an interactive component existed—when the audience was asked to participate. For the interactive events, there was an average "vitality effect" of 2.5 cm (the scale was 10 cm long). A movie on the other hand had a very small vitality effect (average 0.5 cm). In both cases, the standard deviation was around 2. This means that there was a strong and highly statistically significant difference between the interactive theatre performance and the movie show among the 40 participants in the study. The jazz event had a powerful joy effect but a relatively small influence on vitality. The movie which had such a small vitality effect on the other hand had a much more pronounced joy effect.

The interesting question whether the effect of passive listening to music is smaller than the effect of performing music leads us to the discussion in the next chapter about music therapy with both active and passive components.

References

Arnetz, B., Theorell, T., Levi, L., Kallner, A., & Eneroth, P. (1983). An experimental study of social isolation of elderly people: Psychoendocrine and metabolic effects. *Psychosomatic Medicine, 45*, 395–406.

Atkinson, G., Wilson, D., & Eubank, M. (2004). Effects of music on work-rate distribution during a cycling time trial. *International Journal of Sports Medicine, 25*(8), 611–615.

Barlett, D. L. (1996). Physiological responses to music and sound stimuli. In D. A. Hodges (Ed.), *Handbook of music psychology* (2nd ed.). San Antonio: IMR Press.

Beeli, G., Esslen, M., & Jäncke, L. (2005). When coloured sounds taste sweet. *Nature, 434*, 38.

Bernardi, L., & Sleight, P. (2007). Music and biological rhythms. In M. Klockars & M. Peltomaa (Eds.), *Music meets medicine. Acta Gyllenbergiana VII.* Helsinki: The Signe and Ane Gyllenberg Foundation.

Bettermann, H., von Bonin, D., Fruwirth, M., Cysarz, D., & Moser, M. (2002). Effects of speech therapy with poetry on heart rate rhythmicity and cardiorespiratory coordination. *International Journal of Cardiology, 84*, 77–88.

Bittman, B. B., Berk, L., Shannon, M., Sharaf, M., Westengard, J., Guegler, K. J., et al. (2005). Recreational music-making modulates the human stress response: A preliminary individualized gene expression strategy. *Medical Science Monitor, 11*(2), BR31.

Bittman, B. B., Snyder, C., Bruhn, K. T., Liebfried, F., Stevens, C. K., Westengard, J., Umbach, P. O. (2004). Recreational music-making: An integrative group intervention for reducing burnout and improving mood states in first year associate degree nursing students: Insights and economic impact. *International Journal of Nursing Education Scholarship 1*(1) (Article12. Epub 2004 Jul 9)

Blood, A. J., & Zatorre, R. J. (2001). Intensely pleasurable responses to music correlate with activity in brain regions implicated in reward and emotion. *Proceedings of the National Academy of Sciences, 98*, 11818–11823.

Boso, M., Politi, P., Barale, F., & Enzo, E. (2006). Neurophysiology and neurobiology of the musical experience. *Functional Neurology, 21*(4), 187–191. Review.

Bygren, L. O., Konlaan, B. B., & Johansson, S. E. (1996). Attendance at cultural events, reading books or periodicals, and making music or singing in a choir as determinant of survival. Swedish fourteen-year cohort follow-up. *British Medical Journal, 313*, 1577–1580.

Bygren, L. O., Johansson, S.-E., Konlaan, B. B., Grjibovski, A. M., Wilkinson, A. V., & Sjöström, M. (2009). Attending cultural events and cancer mortality: A Swedish cohort study arts & health. *An International Journal for Research Policy and Practice, 1*, 64–73.

Chen, D. D., Xu, X., Zhao, Q., Yin, J., Sallam, H., & Chen, J. D. (2005). Alteration of gastric myoelectrical and autonomic activities with audio stimulation in healthy humans. *Scandinavian Journal of Gastroenterology, 40*(7), 814–821.

Copeland, B. L., & Franks, B. D. (1991). Effects of types and intensities of background music on treadmill endurance. *The Journal of Sports Medicine and Physical Fitness, 31*(1), 100–103.

Daoussis, L., & Mc Kelvie, S. J. (1986). Musical preferences and effects of music on a reading comprehension test for extraverts and introverts. *Perceptual and Motor Skills, 62*, 283–289.

Fagius, J. (2002). *Hemisfärernas musik.* Uppsala: Bo Ejeby förlag.

Gabrielsson, A. (2011). *Strong experiences with music: Music is much more than just music.* Oxford: Oxford University Press.

Hartzell, M., Theorell, T. (2007). Regelbundet återkommande kulturella aktiviteter på arbetsplatsen. Regularly occurring cultural activities in the workplace. National Institute for Psychosocial Factors and Health, p. 2665, Stockholm.

Juslin, P. N., & Sloboda, J. A. (2013). Music and emotion. In D. Deutsch (Ed.), *The psychology of music* (3rd ed., pp. 583–645). Amsterdam: Elsevier.

Khalfa, S., Bella, S. D., Roy, M., Peretz, I., & Lupien, S. J. (2003). Effects of relaxing music on salivary cortisol level after psychological stress. *Annals of the New York Academy of Sciences, 999*, 374–376.

Krantz, G., Madison, G., & Merker, B. (2006). Melodic intervals as reflected in body movement. In *Ninth International Conference on Music Perception and Cognition*, Bologna August 22–26, 2006

Krantz, G., Kreutz, G., Ericson, M., & Theorell, T. (2010). Bodily movements influence heart rate variability (HRV) responses to isolated melodic intervals. *Music and Medicine, 3*(2), 108–113.

Krumhansl, C. L. (1997). An exploratory study of musical emotions and psychophysiology. *Canadian Journal of Experimental Psychology, 51*, 336–352.

Körlin, D. (2005). Creative arts therapy in psychiatry: A clinical application of the Bonny method of guided imagery and music and creative arts groups. Academic thesis, Karolinska Institute, Stockholm.

Le Doux, J. (1998). *The emotional brain*. New York: Weidenfeld and Nicolson.

Lingham, J., & Theorell, T. (2009). Self-selected "favourite" stimulative and sedative music listening—How does familiar and preferred music listening affect the body? *Nordic Journal of Music Therapy, 18*, 150–166.

Panksepp, J. (1995). The emotional sources of "chills" induced by music. *Music Perception, 13*, 171–207.

Rider, M. S., Achterberg, J., Lawlis, G. F., Goven, A., Toledo, R., & Butler, J. R. (1990). Effect of immune system imagery on secretory IgA. *Biofeedback and Self-Regulation, 15*, 317–333.

Szmedra, L., & Bacharach, D. W. (1998). Effect of music on perceived exertion, plasma lactate, norepinephrine and cardiovascular hemodynamics during treadmill running. *International Journal of Sports Medicine, 19*, 32–37.

Väänänen, A., Murray, M., Koskinen, A., Vahtera, J., Kouvonen, A., & Kivimäki, M. (2009). Engagement in cultural activities and cause-specific mortality: Prospective cohort study. *Preventive Medicine, 49*, 142–147.

Vickhoff, B., Åström, R., Theorell, T., von Scheele, B., & Nilsson, M. (2012). Musical piloerection. *Music and Medicine, 4*, 82–89.

Vickhoff, B. (2008). A perspective theory of music perception and emotion. Skrifter från musikvetenskap, Göteborgs universitet, nr 90, ISBN 978 91-85974-06-1, ISSN 1654-6261.

Chapter 6
Music in Treatment

The most common idea about music in treatment is that music has a calming effect and that this is therapeutic. According to this idea a calming effect is what a patient needs. In line with this, there is market for calming music for people with different kinds of psychological and medical problems. This is, however, a very simplified idea of what music can be used for in treatment. The most advanced use of music in treatment is formalised music therapy. Education in music therapy is offered at many universities around the world. It is mostly organised as a specific branch of education within colleges of music and invites trained musicians who have previously acquired competence in psychotherapy. Serving as a music therapist requires extensive knowledge both in music and in psychotherapy. I am not a music therapist myself. I feel deep respect for the double competence that music therapists have. Most music therapists are active in psychiatry. Consequently, most of the patients who receive music therapy are psychiatric patients or subjects with psychological problems. However, music interventions can be used also in somatic conditions, for instance chronic pain. And if we extend our discussion to situations in which we try to improve health, we can see for instance that music can be used in the gym and in dementia care for the benefit of both staff and patients.

In health care, there is insufficient insight into the extensive areas in which music interventions can be used. With sufficient such insight, we would have had many more students in music therapy. At present, there are few students, and in addition, licensed music therapists have difficulties to find a job.

The underlying principle in music therapy is that the emotional state that the patient needs in order to make progress should be induced or amplified (see for instance Bonny 1978; Grönlund et al. 1999; Ruud 1998; Engström 1998; Paulander 2011). If the patient needs to get angry in order to obtain energy to take steps to change his or her life, the music should induce or amplify anger. In the same vein, some patients need to admit that they feel sadness because of something that should be mourned. Other patients may need music that makes them proud and improves their assertiveness. Accordingly, the therapist should have extensive knowledge in what types of music that could be used for strengthening

T. Theorell, *Psychological Health Effects of Musical Experiences*,
SpringerBriefs in Psychology, DOI: 10.1007/978-94-017-8920-2_6,

various emotional states as well as good training in psychotherapy so that he or she can see “where the patient is situated” in a psychological process. A serious aspect is that the consequences of a musical experience are hard to predict. This is true also of other cultural experiences. It means that a strong musical experience can trigger violent and uncontrollable psychological processes in persons with psychological problems. Music therapy is therefore something for music therapists. The therapist must be able to take care of the reactions that are induced. In addition, in particular when the patient has a serious illness requiring long lasting treatment, the therapist needs the backing of an organisation or a supervisor able to help him or her identify his or her own reactions in order to see the patient’s psychological process in a wide perspective.

A form of music therapy that has been used mainly in psychiatry is GIM (Guided Imagery and Music). It has several subtypes of which one is the Bonny method. The Association of Music and Imagery (AMI) officially defines the Bonny Method of Guided Imagery and Music (GIM) as

> a music-centred exploration of consciousness. It offers persons the opportunity to integrate mental, emotional, physical, and spiritual aspects of well-being, as well as awaken to a greater transcendent identity. It is practiced primarily in psychotherapy and counselling settings. Specially sequenced classical music programs are used to stimulate and sustain a dynamic unfolding of inner experiences. Specially sequenced classical music programs are used to stimulate and sustain a dynamic unfolding of inner experiences (for a discussion see Maack 2012).

A Bonny method GIM session starts with a “preliminary” conversation, in which the therapist assesses the patient’s mood, energy level and level of vulnerability in order to arrive at a proper choice of music. This is followed by the patient’s listening to the music that the therapist selected doing this in a comfortable relaxing position. During listening, the patient is asked to imagine pictures. In the post-session, the therapist and the patient process the thoughts and pictures together and try to relate them to the patient’s life situation. GIM can be used both in individual therapy and in groups. And it can be used work with healthy people as well (Wrangsjö and Körlin 1995).

A recently published study has shown that 50 sessions of the Bonny method GIM is therapeutically useful for patients with complex post-traumatic stress disorder (Maack 2012). In this context, “complex” means that the patient has had not only one but several difficult psychic trauma(ta) and that this gives rise to a therapeutically particularly difficult situation. The study also indicates that the GIM therapy has better effects than Psychodynamic Imaginative Trauma Therapy, a treatment somewhat similar to GIM but without music. Significant improvement after GIM has also been shown in psychiatric disorders by Körlin (2005) in controlled evaluations.

Another study (McKinney et al. 1997) showed that subjects who were participating in GIM sessions had decreasing salivary cortisol levels during wake hours, as a possible indicator of decreased habitual arousal levels during the daily round of life.

There are several forms of music therapy, some of which build upon psychodynamic principles and some on salutogenesis and positive psychology (resource-oriented music therapy). The main point in the salutogenic approach is that the therapy should help the patient or client identify his/her own strength. For a more extensive discussion, see Rolvsjord (2010). Ruud (1998) has discussed whether or not theoretical verbal analysis of music communication in individual therapy is important. It could be argued that music's strong effects do not need to be explained in psychological verbal terms in the individual case. For further discussion, see also Paulander (2011).

Music therapy (and other kinds of music interventions) could have both "passive" (to listen) and "active" (to make music or sound, often together with the therapist) components. The active components should be constructed in such a way that the patient is not asked to be a "clever" musician. There should be no musical achievement demands, and no musical evaluation. In the more advanced forms of music therapy, there is access to several musical instruments, including drums. A skilful therapist can create a powerful emotional atmosphere, and since the patient is actively contributing to the sound, the effect may be quite strong. In a therapeutic programme that we were running, the Art Psychotherapeutic Programme (Theorell et al. 1998), our patients had chronic pain and at the same time other psychosomatic conditions which had resulted in working incapacity since at least two years. They were attending therapy once a week for two years, and they were allocated to one out of four possible therapies, namely dance, music, painting and theatre. The allocation was based upon our assessment of what would be the most useful therapy for them and professionals were not allocated to their own type of art—no musician to music, for instance. The therapists worked as a group with patient-centred meetings once every two weeks and this meant that a patient in music therapy might have drawn pictures that were shown to the therapist group and the therapeutic course could be discussed jointly. The four therapists were supplemented with a physician who had the medical responsibility (myself) and a psychologist who had the psychotherapeutic responsibility (Konarski).

The main task in the evaluation of the Art Psychotherapeutic Programme was to describe "turning points" in the therapeutic courses. The music therapist (Engström) described one such important turning point. A woman aged 42 with severe chronic back pain had been attending music therapy in the programme for several weeks. During the session, the therapist intended to create a threatening atmosphere. Both the therapist and the patient used a big drum and they started together drumming an aggressive "war rhythm". The patient became increasingly engaged in this and was finally totally absorbed. After a while, she interrupted herself exhausted and sweating with the following statement: Oh: I do not have any pain now!

It is not strange that our patient did not experience any pain in this engaged and absorbed moment. It could be that her blood concentration of endorphin, the body's own morphine, increased, which is often the case during pronounced arousal. The pain returned after some time (when the endorphin concentration had decreased?). However, she had not experienced a painless state for a very long time. Now she saw that she might have a life without pain again. This insight was very positive for her continued clinical course. The threatening rhythm had another influence. It brought back memories of incest experiences that she had had during her childhood. She saw disgusting pictures that she was asked to draw pictures of. These pictures could then be used in her therapy. This woman was intensively engaged in the music therapy in several other ways. She listened energetically to the music and participated in great zest in music making with the therapist during the sessions.

There were other components in our evaluation. The patients were asked to fill in standardised symptom questionnaires approximately once every fourth month. On these occasions, venous blood samples were collected. These were analysed with regard to chemical substances that mirror stress and regeneration. The typical course in these patients who came to us in a relatively passive state due to their chronic pain was the following:

Biologically most patients showed a low energy level at start. During the first weeks, the patient and the therapist were exploring together crucial experiences that may have been of significance to explain their state. After approximately half a year, there was often a dramatic cultural experience ("turning point" as mentioned above). During this period, the energy level (in this study mirrored by the blood concentration of uric acid, which is known to increase during periods of increased energy) increased. Then came a period of resolution and calm during which the energy level decreased again. Unfortunately, the regenerative and anabolic activities in the body, mirrored in the concentration of DHEA-s, a steroid hormone with such activity, was low in this patient group, and there was no significant evidence of regenerative improvement in the total group during the two-year study period. However, the mental state (degree of anxiety and depression) had improved significantly in most patients during the first year. Their quality of life improved in the sense that they had become socially more active after two years. In addition, their working capacity improved. In many, but not all, cases, the somatic symptoms had decreased after two years.

There were pronounced differences between the patients during the two study years, and in some cases, strong effects were observed, whereas only very small effects were observed in other cases. For the woman whose "turning point" was described above, there were several effects, both somatic and psychological. Figure 6.1 shows how the assessed variables changed during a two-year period. As in most clinical, longitudinal studies, there are occasional missing data on some observation points. In the diagram, the starting point for each variable has been set at 1.0, and all changes on the y axis are expressed as ratios indicating the ratio between the observed value at follow-up and the starting point. The only exception from this is self-rated health (red in the diagram), which the patient has been asked to rate on a five-grade scale. The number 1 corresponds to poor self-rated health and 5 to excellent. The patient reported poor health, as did most patients in the study, during the first 15 months after which improvement is seen. The level of anxiety and depressive symptoms (blue) is elevated during the first ten months but then oscillates around the initial level. The green line corresponds to serum uric acid, and it mirrors energy level. The diagram shows an increased level during the initial 15–20-month period after which a decrease is seen (see above). Serum

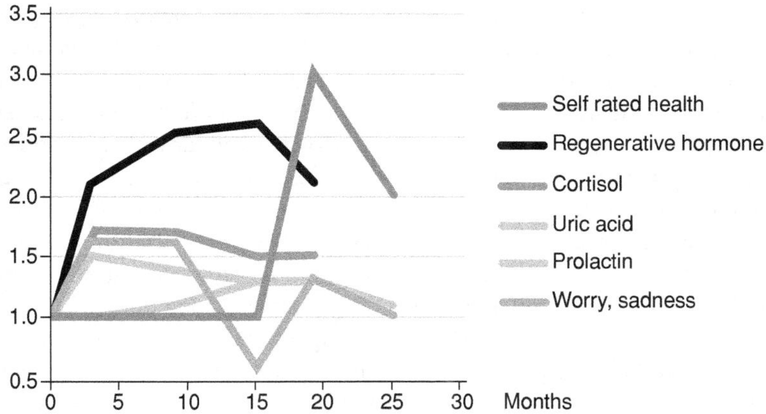

Fig. 6.1 Engaged patient, blood concentration and self-reported health scores. All levels are related to the starting level which is equal to 1

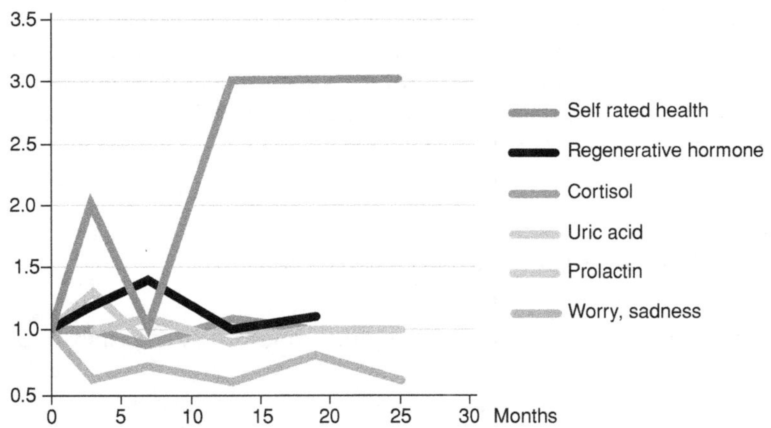

Fig. 6.2 Disengaged patient, blood concentration and self-reported health scores. All levels are related to the starting level which is equal to 1

cortisol (light blue) is also reflecting energy level but has a more rapid response pattern than uric acid. It has its peak level five to ten months from start and then decreases but never down to the low starting level. In this patient, the blood concentration of the regenerative hormone DHEA-s (black) increases considerably during the study period. It reaches its peak 15 months after start but is still doubled after 20 months. Serum prolactin (grey) that tends to increase in stress situations which the person lacks control over shows a small increase during the whole study period with an initial peak already during the first months.

For a comparison, I have displayed the corresponding diagram (Fig. 6.2) from another patient attending music therapy in the same study. She was not at all as engaged in her music therapy as the first patient. It could even be argued that she was allocated to the wrong kind of art psychotherapy, she might have been better off in the picture drawing group for instance. To some extent, she even disliked music, particularly when she was asked to make music herself. This diagram is very different from Fig. 6.1. This patient shows hardly any changes during the two-year study period. The only variable that changes is self-rated health (red). In line with this, there is a reduction in anxiety and depressive symptoms.

The two examples show that the individual attitude to music may—not unexpectedly—have an important role in determining effects. Like in all treatments, practice should take both individual and context into consideration.

The most important task in the use of art experiences in rehabilitation and psychotherapy is to help the patient or client find new ways of expressing his or her life situation. Non-verbal methods are essential. A non-verbal art therapy that is close to music therapy is dance therapy. The potential of dance therapy to make patients express feelings that they have had difficulties in expressing before has been described by several authors, for instance by Thulin (2007) and by Bojner Horwitz (2004). Dance therapy is almost always accompanied by music and is one example of a situation in which it is impossible to disentangle the "independent" effect of dance or music. These activities very often occur at the same time and they may even be "programmed" together in our brains. Psychodrama and art (pictures) therapy are also established as therapies supplementing rehabilitation (see Grönlund, Alm and Hammarlund 1999).

Other Music Interventions in Health Care

Music interventions are used increasingly in various kinds of health care. Some examples will follow:

Music listening is used to an increasing extent before (for instance Miluk-Kolasa et al. 1994) and after surgery. RCT (Randomised Controlled Trial) studies in which some patients are allocated to music listening and some of them to silent relaxation have been performed. Such studies have shown decreased pain ratings and decreased consumption of analgesics (pain killing medication) in the music listening groups (Nilsson et al. 2001, 2003; Good et al. 2005). This line of research has also shown that music listening in this situation is associated with a decrease in the blood concentration of cortisol, an indicator of stress reactions that may delay healing of wounds after the operation. In addition, it has been shown that patients who wake up from heart surgery have an increased blood concentration of oxytocin whereas those who wake up in silence have a decrease during the same period (Nilsson 2009). This is important because oxytocin has been shown to decrease pain and anxiety. In a similar vein, patients undergoing the C clamp procedure after percutaneous coronary interventions (Chan et al. 2006), widening of narrowed coronary vessels without open-heart surgery, have participated in an RCT with/without music listening. Results 45 min after the coronary intervention showed that the music listening group had reduced pain whereas the control group had increased pain. Similarly four indices of stress (heart rate, blood pressure, respiratory rate and oxygen saturation) had reduced levels after surgery whereas no such reduction was observed in the control group.

In all acute health care situations such as surgery and non-surgical coronary interventions, it is important that the music listening is individualised. Ulrica Nilsson, who has been doing extensive studies on the effects of music listening, has discussed this emphasising that in the beginning, she and her collaborators were playing too complicated music. The selection of musical pieces has to be individualised, and it should be based upon a discussion between the health care staff and the patient. A "musical menu" of cd recordings (or similar recordings) should be available—as on long-distance flights. In addition, it is important that the listening equipment is adequate and adapted to the patient's particular situation. The sound could be coming from a small pillow for instance. This type of music listening may be important not only for the patients themselves but also for the caring staff who will get calmer patients!

Pain relief is another scientifically documented useful area in which music listening can contribute. The biological mechanism underlying the fact that pain often diminishes with (appropriately adjusted) music listening during or after painful medical interventions is unknown. What has been shown in a small number of studies is that the stress-related rise in cortisol concentration vanishes faster with music than with silence, so it is likely that reduction of stress may play a role here. Cepeda et al. (2006) have summarised the literature in this field concluding that music intervention does have significant albeit small pain-relieving effects. This confirms an early review published by Standley (1995). The conclusion that the effect is small albeit significant has been criticised on the basis that Cepeda's review did not include interventions comprising both music listening and hypnotic suggestion. This is a combination that is particularly effective according to some authors (see Hanser 2006).

Music listening and participation in musical activities are also used in *oncological care*. Music therapy can be used as an aid for patients to overcome the dramatic trauma that the onset of cancer illness means. Music therapy can in general improve the quality of life for these patients. As pointed out by Olofsson and Fossum (2009), underlying scientific concepts have varied greatly in this field. But there is agreement that music therapy has great potential in oncological care.

> The music therapist assesses the patient and consults other members of the multidisciplinary team to create a therapeutic treatment plan. Music therapists design music sessions based on patients' needs and their intended therapeutic goals. Patients can participate actively or passively in individual or group sessions. Only a credentialed music therapist can provide safe and beneficial music therapy interventions (Mahon and Mahon 2011; see also Bradt et al. (2011) and Daykin et al. (2007).

Care of demented patients is an important application area for musical activities. Severely, demented patients often lack orientation with regard to space, time and person. This also means that feeding and clothing them could be difficult for the caring staff because the patient may feel threatened. He or she may bite, shout and spit in order to show unwillingness to cooperate. It has been discovered (Götell 2000) that singing for (and sometimes with) the patient may alleviate the tension. In particular, songs that bear a relationship to the patient's early years (for instance Ba Ba Black Sheep) may have a calming effect. And the effect is not only calming; the patient all of a sudden seems to understand the situation and cooperates much more willingly. In addition, he/she may turn out to be known the song's words and tune even better than the staff.

A related area is music intervention in care of patients with *stroke or other brain damage resulting in aphasia*. The patient may not be able to tell people in the environment when he/she is hungry. It has been shown, however, (Myskja 2006a) that many patients in this situation may be able to sing the words I am hungry to the staff even when they cannot speak the words. Simple tunes should be used in the instruction, for instance aaab (I am hungry) where b is a minor third lower than a (same tune as priests are singing during the sermon when they are introducing a prayer).

A Finnish group of researchers (Särkämö et al. 2008) has shown that music listening can accelerate the *healing process after a stroke*. That study was also an RCT study. 60 patients with stroke due to occlusion of one of the brain arteries participated. They were randomly allocated to three groups. One group listened to individually selected taped music, a second group listened to taped novel reading and a third group did not listen to any tape. At follow-up two months after start, the patients in the music group had improved significantly more than the other patients with regard to memory and ability to concentrate. Although more similar studies are needed this study indicates that music listening, if adjusted in a proper way to the situation, may be a neurologically more beneficial than talking.

An additional neurological area in which music listening has been used therapeutically is the treatment of *Parkinson's disease*. Sacks (1997) and Myskja (2006b) have described patients who have pronounced stiffness and lack of ability to coordinate movements to the extent that they are almost unable to walk. When certain types of rhythms are played, their movements are softened and improved coordination is observed. Some of these patients may even turn out to be able to dance when the music is on! A strictly controlled study showed that there was a significant effect of music therapy on these patients (Pacchetti et al. 2000).

Mental retardation is a known field for music interventions. There are examples of groups of subjects with abnormally developed brain function who benefit more than others from the use of music in educational efforts. One such example is subjects with Williams syndrome, a neurogenetic developmental disorder characterised by an increased affinity for music, deficits in verbal memory, and atypical brain development. In two studies, patients who had participated in formal music lessons scored significantly better on the verbal memory task when the sentences were sung than when they were spoken (Martens et al. 2011). Subjects with Williams syndrome are very engaged in music and sometimes develop unusual musical skills and react in unusual ways to music—which is important both positively and negatively in social contacts with them (see Levitin 2005; Järvinen et al. 2012). The ability to appreciate music and to participate in musical activity varies across different groups of subjects with mental retardation. Three- to four-year-old subjects with Down's syndrome, for instance, have been shown to be as able to grasp rhythm as normal children (Stratford and Ching 1983) and therefore benefit greatly from participating in musical activities in groups.

Autistic children and adults (whose main handicap is not mental retardation but difficulty to communicate socially) may benefit substantially from music education. This may make it possible for these persons to get into emotional contact with the environment—something that may be impossible otherwise. Paul Robertson, a British violinist and professor of musicology specialising on music neurology often presents video recordings of such a patient in his lectures (www.musicmindspirit.org). The mother of this boy is a piano teacher and she discovered that she could communicate emotions with him in piano playing. This triggered an important development in the boy's life since he developed considerable skill in piano playing and was able to illustrate a broad repertoire of emotions by playing them. It also contributed to an improved general development of his life.

Sleeping difficulties. Music listening is also discussed in relation to sleep disorders. A recent experimental study showed for instance that regular music listening with special equipment was associated with subjectively improved sleep although objective indicators (EEG) did not show any improvement (Harmat et al. 2008).

What the benefits of music interventions in neurological and developmental difficulties may illustrate is that the brains of these groups of subjects do not function in the same way as the majority of brains. Some connections in their brain have been broken or have never existed. When the environment tries to reach vital brain functions, the "usual" methods, for instance rational verbal arguments, do not work, but somewhere deep inside the brain, the functions are there. The challenge is to find out how to reach them. Music activates the brain in other ways than the rational verbal argument. Referring again to Le Doux and his research (see Chap. 5), both auditory and visual impulses reach the brain via a "high" and a "low" route. Many of the impulses from music are rapidly transferred directly to the emotional brain via the "low" (and fast) route. From there, it is possible that the impulses are spread via "backstage" impulses to the brain centres that cannot be reached the "usual" way.

The integration of the "low" (fast) route to the emotional brain and the "high" (slow) route to the brain cortex is of decisive importance in psychosomatic illness. If the individual is unable to identify and interpret different kinds of emotional impulses because this ability has not been developed or damaged, this person suffers from *alexithymia.* This could of course be more or less advanced. In its most extreme form, all feelings ranging from happiness to sadness and anger are unidentified, and this creates difficulties with social interaction and self-regulation in stressful situations. Alexithymia increases the risk of developing psychosomatic illnesses (for instance high blood pressure, see Theorell 2012). The underlying psychological mechanism this is probably that a correct interpretation of an emotional reaction serves as guidance in stressful situations. The person who does not know whether he or she is angry, sad or anxious is disoriented. Instead of finding guidance in the emotion, the person may remain in a vague feeling of uneasiness without knowing what to do. If this feeling is long lasting and often repeated, such unsolved situations may give rise to psychophysiological reactions increasing the risk for instance of cardiovascular disease (Grabe et al. 2010).

The discussion regarding alexithymia provides important support for helping children develop a good ability to identify and interpret their own feelings. Musical activities in the family and at school could stimulate this. Emotional ability may be decisive for these individuals when they become adults and may also be one of the factors contributing to a healthy development in a life perspective. This is discussed more extensively in Chap. 9. (See also Smith 2005.) But the principle that music may activate the brain in other ways than rational verbal argumentation may also explain why music therapy may add substantially to psychotherapy. Unexpected emotional experiences, arising in a specific context where the musical stimulus adds to the situation, may activate the brain in such a way that the patient starts looking at his or her life in a new way. This principle may explain why music therapy may add to the results of rehabilitation (see above) or to choir singing (see Chap. 8). An unblocked musical stimulus may give rise to re-evaluation (perhaps a new perspective on a rigid super-ego??) which changes the future life course. Gabrielsson (2011) has performed more than a thousand interviews with subjects who were asked to describe in their own words their strongest musical experience ever. This study supports the profound importance that music has in evoking strong feelings with long-term effects. Several individuals describe how a strong musical experience has changed their life.

I mentioned the possibility that, once the emotional reaction has activated the emotional brain, there may be an activation of other parts of the brain via alternative routes. This may for instance explain the sudden moment of clarity described above in the severely demented patient when a child song is sung. Links between brain cells handling interpretation of the spoken words and memory cells helping orientation may have been broken due to the brain disease. But when the musical stimulus activates the emotional brain, impulses may find their way "backstage", activating memories that are still intact but mainly unused because they have been cut off. Emotional memories are of course not only negative (sad, angry and anxious) but also positive (proud, happy and curious). The potential use of cultural experiences in alternative brain activation could also be applied to non-musical cultural experiences with strong non-verbal components (pictures, dance, some kinds of sports, etc.).

A special form of music therapy is the Tomatis treatment (Sinha et al. 2011). This treatment introduced by a French physician builds upon extensive listening to classical pieces of music that have been fragmented and changed. The effects obtained are probably due to mechanisms discussed above—that brain centres that are hard to communicate with when verbal arguments are used become more available and that the fragmented music functions as a training instrument for the brain cells. In individual cases, striking effects have been reported in autism and some other neurological and psychiatric conditions (including the burnout syndrome). Strong scientific support, however, is still lacking (Sinha et al. 2011), according to a recent Cochrane report. Those who administer the treatment have been criticised because they have not explained the underlying principles behind the fragmentation of the music.

Therapeutic music may also be individually tailored. First of all, information is gathered about the patient's musical preferences and previous experiences and the team then composes individually tailored music. Secondly this music could be switched on when the body is particularly beneficially receptive to it. Brandes et al. (2009) have examined the effects of music intervention following both principles. In a four-arm randomised, placebo- and waiting-list-controlled double-blind study, including 150 participants, two specific music programmes significantly reduced burnout symptoms after 5 weeks. The effects were maintained over a long-time period. In the same study, reduction in depressive symptoms was shown as well (Brandes et al. 2010). The same group (Brandes et al. 2008) has also shown that it is possible to stimulate the activity of the parasympathetic system by means of these highly individualised music programmes. If patients with high blood pressure participate in such treatment programmes for extended periods, it may be possible also to reduce blood pressure since activation of the parasympathetic system reduces heart rate and blood pressure.

Although there are exceptions, most of the utilisation of music in treatments builds upon passive consumption. In the next chapter, I shall discuss how active music making, singing, affects the body.

References

Bojner Horwitz, E. (2004). Dance/movement therapy in fibromyalgia patients: Aspects and consequences of verbal, visual and hormonal analyses. Doctoral thesis. Acta Universitatis Upsaliensis, Uppsala University.

Bonny, H. L. (1978). *Facilitating guided imagery and music sessions*. Baltimore: ICM Books.

Bradt, J., Cileo, C., Grocke, D., & Magill, L. (2011). Music interventions for improving psychological and physical outcomes in cancer patients (review). Cochrane Dabaser of Systematic Reviews (8). Art. No.: CD006911. doi:10.1002/14651858.CD006911.pub2.

Brandes, V., Terris, D. D., Fischer, C., Schuessler, M. N., Ottowitz, G., Titscher, G., et al. (2009). Music programs designed to remedy burnout symptoms show significant effects after five weeks. *Annals of the New York Academy of Sciences, 1169*, 422–425.

Brandes, V., Terris, D. D., Fischer, C., Loerbroks, A., Jarczok, M. N., Ottowitz, G., et al. (2010). Receptive music therapy for the treatment of depression: a proof-of-concept study and prospective controlled clinical trial of efficacy. *Psychotherapy and Psychosomatics, 79*(5), 321–322.

Brandes, V., Thayer, J. & Fischer, J.E. (2008). The effect of receptive music therapy on heart rate variability in hypertensive patients. Scientific Poster at the Annual Meeting of the American Psychosomatic Society, Baltimore.

Cepeda, M.S., Carr, D.B., Lau, J., & Alvarez, H. (2006). Music for pain relief. Cochrane Database of Systematic Reviews 2006, (2). Art. No.:CD004843. doi:10.1001/146651858. CD004843.pub2.

Chan, M. F., Wong, O. C., Chan, H. L., Fong, M. C., Lai, S. Y., Lo, C. W., et al. (2006). Effects of music on patients undergoing a C-clamp procedure after percutaneous coronary interventions. *Journal of Advanced Nursing, 53*(6), 669–679.

Daykin, N., Mc Clean, S., & Bunt, L. (2007). Creativity, identity and healing: Participants' accounts of music therapy in cancer care. *Health, 11*, 349–370.

Engström, R. (1998). Musikterapi (Music therapy). In T. Theorell (red.), När orden inte räcker. (When words are not enough) Natur och Kultur, Stockholm.

Gabrielsson, A. (2011). *Strong experiences with music—music is much more than just music*. Oxford: Oxford University Press.

Good, M., Anderson, G. C., Ahn, S., Cong, X., & Stanton-Hicks, M. (2005). Relaxation and music reduce pain following intestinal surgery. *Research in Nursing & Health, 28*(3), 240–251.

Grabe, H.J., Schwahn, C., Barnow, S., Spitzer, C., John, U., Freyberger, H.J., Schminke, U., Felix, S., & Völzke, H. (2010). Alexithymia, hypertension, and subclinical atherosclerosis in the general population. Journal of Psychosomatic Research. *68*(2), 139–147. doi:10.1016/j.jpsychores.2009.07.015 (epub 17 Nov 2009).

Grönlund, E., Alm, A., & Hammarlund, I. (1999). Bild, dans och musik i den läkande processen. (Visual arts, dance and music in healing processes) Natur och Kultur, Stockholm.

Götell, E., Brown, S., & Ekman, S.-L. (2000). Caregiver-assisted music events in psychogeriatric care. *Journal of Psychiatric and Mental Health Nursing, 7*, 119–125.

Hanser, S. B. (2006). Music therapy research in adult oncology. *Journal of the Society for Integrative Oncology, 4*(2), 62–66.

Harmat, L, de Manzano, Ö., Theorell, T., Ullén, F. (2013). The psychophysiology of optimal experience: Parasympathetic activation is higher during flow states than during effortful attention. In review 2012, Department of Neuroscience, Karolinska Institute.

Harmat, L., Takacs, J., & Bodizs, R. (2008). Music improves sleep quality. *Journal of Advanced Nursing, 62*, 327–335.

Järvinen, A., Dering, B., Neumann, D., Ng, R., Crivelli, D., Grichanik, M., Korenberg, J.R., Bellugi, U. (2012). Sensitivity of the autonomic nervous system to visual and auditory affect across social and non-social domains in Williams syndrome. Frontiers in Psychology *3*, 343. doi:10.3389/fpsyg.2012.00343 (epub 14 Sep 2012).

Körlin, D. (2005). Creative arts therapy in psychiatry: A clinical application of the Bonny method of guided imagery and music and creative arts groups. Akademisk avhandling, Karolinska Institutet, Stockholm.

Levitin, D. J. (2005). Musical behaviour in a neurogenetic developmental disorder: evidence from Williams Syndrome. *Annals of the New York Academy of Sciences, 1060*, 325–334.

Maack, C. (2012). Outcomes and processes of the Bonny Method of guided imagery and music and its adaptations and psychodynamic imaginative trauma therapy for women with complex PTSD. Department of Communication and Psychology. University of Aalborg, Denmark.

Mahon, E.M., Mahon S.M. (2011). Music therapy: a valuable adjunct in the oncology setting. *Clinical Journal of Oncology Nursing, 15*(4), 353–356. doi:10.1188/11.CJON.353-356.

Martens, M. A., Jungers, M. K., & Steele, A. L. (2011). Effect of musical experience on verbal memory in Williams Syndrome: Evidence from a novel word learning task. *Neuropsychologia, 49*, 3093–3102.

McKinney, C. H., Antoni, M. H., Kumar, M., Tims, F. C., & McCabe, P. M. (1997). Effects of guided imagery and music (GIM) therapy on mood and cortisol in healthy adults. *Health Psychology, 16*, 390–400.

Miluk-Kolasa, B., Obminski, Z., Stupnicki, R., Golec, L. (1994). Effects of music treatment on salivary cortisol in patients exposed to pre-surgery stress. *Experimental and Clinical Endocrinology, 102*, 118–120.

Myskja, A. (2006b). Å finne rytmen (To find the rhythm). Oslo: Norges Parkinsonforbund.

Myskja, A. (2006a). Den musiske medisin (Music Medicine) Oslo Cappelen.

Nilsson, U. (2009). Soothing music can increase oxytocin levels during bed rest after open heart surgery in "Music" versus "Control" group: a randomized control trial. *Journal of Clinical Nursing, 18*, 2153–2161.

Nilsson, U., Rawal, N., & Unosson, M. (2003). A comparison of intra-operative or postoperative exposure to music—a controlled trial of the effect on postoperative pain. *Anaesthesia, 58*, 673–699.

Nilsson, U., Rawal, N., Unestahl, L. E., Zetterberg, C., & Unosson, M. (2001). Improved recovery after music and therapeutic suggestions during general anaesthesia: a double-blind randomised controlled trial. *Acta Anaesthesiologica Scandinavica, 45*(7), 812–817.

Olofsson, A., & Fossum, B. (2009). Perspectives on music therapy in adult cancer care: A hermeneutic study. *Oncology Nursing Forum, 36*(4), E223–E231. doi:10.1188/09.ONF. E223-E231.Review.

Pacchetti, C., Mancini, F., Aglieri, R., Fundaro, C., Martignoni, E., & Nappi, G. (2000). Active music therapy in Parkinson's disease: An integrative method for motor and emotional rehabilitation. Psychosomatic Medicine, *62*(3), 386–993.

Paulander, A.-S. (2011). Meningen med att gå i musikterapi (Meaning of attending music therapy). Doctoral thesis, Royal College of Music, Stockholm, Sweden.

Rolvsjord, R. (2010). *Resource-oriented music therapy in mental health care.* Gilsum: Barcelona Publishers.

Ruud, E. (1998). *Music therapy: Improvisation, communication and culture.* Gilsum: Barcelona Publishers.

Sinha, Y., Silove, N., Hayen, A., Williams, K. (2011). Auditory integration training and other sound therapies for autism spectrum disorders (ASD). Cochrane Database of Systematic Reviews, (12):CD003681. doi:10.1002/14651858.CD003681.pub3. (Review).

Stratford, B., & Ching, E. Y. (1983). Rhythm and time in the perception of Down's syndrome children. *Journal of Mental Deficiency Research, 27*, 23–38.

Sacks, O. (1997). Island of the colorblind. Paperback, Vintage Books, ISBN 0-375-70073-0.

Särkämö, T., Tervaniemi, M., Laitinen, S., Forsblom, A., Soinila, S., Mikkonen, M., et al. (2008). Music listening enhances cognitive recovery and mood after middle cerebral artery stroke. *Brain, 131*, 866–876.

Smith, G. (2005). Estetisk perception på emotionell botten (Aesthetic perception on emotional basis). In Hermerén G (red): Konsterna och själen. Estetik ur ett humanvetenskapligt perspektiv. (The arts and the soul. Aesthetics from a humanistic percpective) Konferens nr 61, Kungl Historie- och Vitterhetsakademien. Stockholm.

Standley, J. (1995). Music as a therapeutic intervention in medical and dental treatment. Research and clinical applications. In T. Wigram, B. Saperston, R. West (Eds.), The art and science of music therapy. A handbook. Switzerland: Harwood Academic Publishers.

Theorell, T., Konarski, K., Westerlund, H., Burell, A.-M., Engström, R., Lagercrantz, A.-M., et al. (1998). Treatment of patients with chronic somatic symptoms by means of art psychotherapy—A process description. *Psychotherapy and Psychosomatics, 67*, 50–56.

Theorell, T. (red). (1998). När orden inte räcker (When words are not enough). Natur och Kultur, Stockholm.

Theorell, T. (2012). Evaluating life events and stressors in relation to health: Stressors and health in clinical work. *Advances in Psychosomatic Medicine, 32*, 58–71.

Thulin, K. (2007). Alla dessa rum. Om skapande, rörelse, lek och dans. (All these rooms. On creativity, movement and dance) Carlssons, Stockholm.

Wrangsjö, B., & Körlin, D. (1995). Guided imagery and music as a psychotherapeutic method in psychiatry. *Journal of the Association for Music and Imagery, 4*, 79–92.

Chapter 7
What Happens in the Body During Singing?

Music in the Body

I often get the question: What happens in the body during singing? It is not so difficult to describe the immediate psychological effects of singing. Most subjects who are asked to describe how they feel after singing describe a feeling of increased energy, and they also feel more relaxed than before singing. But there is considerable variation. The experience depends to a great extent on previous experiences of singing: The mere thought of singing may make some people sweat and even feel "scared to death". Previous experiences have been both somatic and psychological and these relate to one another in a complicated way. It is more difficult to understand the effects of singing than to understand the effects of music listening. This is of course due to the fact that singing engages the body in a particular way that affects breathing, cardiovascular functions and hormones. Accordingly, the only thing we can do is mostly to describe the "total" effect of singing. It is almost impossible to know whether the effects that we observe are due to aesthetic experiences and emotional reactions to these or to bodily processes associated with the physical production of the singing sounds. During later years, an increasing number of scientific publications have discussed bodily effects of singing and almost all of them deal with the immediate effects. In these studies, psychological states as well as effects on hormonal systems, on immunological and cardiovascular functions as well as on other biological stress parameters (such as sweating) have been assessed.

The most frequently assessed physiological parameter in studies of singing is heart rate. Elevated heart rate mirrors a state of arousal, a high "body speed". I will therefore discuss how much heart rate change may be associated with singing and what conditions that may influence this change.

It is also possible, however, to derive more complex information from recorded variations in heart rate, so-called HRV (heart rate variability). Due to the development of advanced technology that can process large amounts of electrocardiographic recordings "online", in this case when people are singing, it has become

T. Theorell, *Psychological Health Effects of Musical Experiences*,
SpringerBriefs in Psychology, DOI: 10.1007/978-94-017-8920-2_7,

Table 7.1 Mean heart rate during ten pairs of music performances (professional flute players and singers)—"strenuous" and "easy" piece with and without audience

Heart rate on average during			
Easy piece		Strenuous piece	
Without audience	With audience	Without audience	With audience
95/m	117/m	99/m	126/m

Source Harmat and Theorell (2010)

possible to analyse factors of importance to the variation itself. It has turned out that these variations contain important information, and they make it possible to analyse the balance between the "accelerating" sympathetic and the "decelerating" parasympathetic nervous system. A high average heart rate during a given time interval may be due either to a high activity in the sympathetic system (SS) or to a low activity in the parasympathetic system (PSS) during that interval. Sometimes the two systems are activated at the same time. HRV tells us more about the respective activities in the two systems than the average heart rate does, mainly because the PSS has a more dominant role in determining HRV than the SS. Of particular importance to singing is the fact that the PSS is sensitive to breathing. Deep slow diaphragm breathing activates the PSS and not only increases HRV but also decreases average heart rate and blood pressure.

A study that was performed in our institute some years ago (Grape et al. 2003) illustrates how different the experience of singing could be. The experimental subjects were eight professional (they were paid part time or full time for their singing) and eight amateur singers. Careful measurements were performed before, during and after a real singing lesson. The study showed that the professionals and the amateurs in several ways reacted differently to this situation both somatically and psychologically, although they also had some reactions in common.

All the participants in the examination of the singing lesson were accustomed to the situation. Even the amateurs should have had at least half a year's experience of taking singing lessons. During normal conditions, a singing lesson is a "safe" situation. Teacher and pupil know one another well and there is no disturbing audience. Although there are strict teachers and scared pupils, they have the same goal, namely to improve the pupil's singing technique. Male and female singers were included in both groups. The age ranged from 25 to 45 years. Before start and after the singing lesson, all participants filled in a short questionnaire, a visual analogue scale (VAS) recording in a simple way three aspects of their emotional state. The visual analogue scale consisted of a 10-cm horizontal line on which the subject was asked to put a cross in the place corresponding to their state in that particular moment. The maximally bad position was located in the left end of the line and the maximally good one in the right end. The three emotional states were the following: maximally sad—maximally joyful, maximally tired—maximally energetic and maximally tense—maximally relaxed. Table 7.1 shows the VAS results before and after the singing lesson.

With regard to the sad–joyful dimension there was no change at all after the singing lesson in the professional singers, whereas the amateurs reported increased joy. Both groups started to the right of the middle of the VAS, i.e. more joyful than sad, but the results showed that the amateurs became even more happy, whereas the professionals stayed on the same level. This professional/amateur group difference in change was statistically significant (two-way analysis of variance). The difference was also obvious in interviews performed after the singing lessons. The singers were asked to describe in their own words how they had perceived their singing lesson. While the amateurs described the joy of singing and how they appreciated the opportunity to enrich their lives, the professionals were obsessed with technical details in their singing and often described it in self-derogatory terms: “Was not able to keep the note long enough”; “Was not in good shape”; “Did not support the notes with my diaphragm”.

For the other two emotional states, tired–energetic and tense–relaxed, however, both groups reported improvements. There was no significant difference between amateurs and professionals from these points of view. Accordingly, the singers became more energetic and more relaxed after the singing lesson regardless of professional status. This particular effect has been described in many other studies, for instance by Sandgren and Borg (2009). These studies were examinations of how “expert” and “non-expert” choir singers experienced a choir rehearsal in Stockholm, a city with many choirs. The pattern observed in this study was that “expert” as well as “non-expert” choir singers showed joy and relaxation during the rehearsals and that there was no striking difference between the groups. The rehearsals are probably “calibrated” to the level of the choir. This may mean that challenges and frustrations may be experienced to the same extent regardless of level of expertise in the choir situation—although for one and the same choir, this will vary across rehearsals depending on repertoire, etc. It will also vary between individuals. But to a great extent, the choir rehearsal is a collective experience. In the individual singing lesson, on the other hand, the professional singer who earns his or her living from performing has to fight for a high-level quality. And there is no doubt that the performance of the voice in the professional differs in several ways from that of the amateur (Sundberg 1989).

According to modern neurobiological research, the brains of professional singers differ from the brains of other people. A neurobiological examination (Kleber et al. 2010) of functional activation in relation to accumulated singing practice has been performed. Highly accomplished opera singers, conservatory level vocal students, and laymen were examined during singing of an Italian aria in a neuroimaging experiment. It showed that singing training increases activation of the parts of the brain that are important for enhanced control of voice muscles and for regulating the sensory function in such muscles. In addition, such training is associated with increased activity in memory areas for these muscles and for the coordination of their movements.

Other research (Wilson et al. 2011) has shown that expert and non-expert singers differ with regard to engagement of the language network in the brain. Non-expert singers engage their brain’s language network to a greater extent than professional singers. These findings indicate that singing expertise promotes independence from the language network, with this "decoupling" producing a more tuneful performance.

Accordingly, we can conclude that professional singing training influences the experience of singing and also changes the brain function in several important ways. But does it also influence cardiovascular function?

First of all, the cardiovascular function is intimately associated with breathing, which is different during singing compared to most other activities. During normal breathing, inhalation and exhalation are of approximately the same duration. Singing on the other hand is characterised by a rapid inhalation and a slow exhalation, the latter also taking place with some resistance because the vocal chords form a narrow passage for the air coming from the lungs. These facts are of importance to the analysis of heart rate variability.

Heart Rate and Heart Rate Variability

During the study of the singing lesson, electrocardiograms were recorded continuously. We observed that the heart rate at rest was normal, between 60 and 80 beats per minute. During singing, the average heart rate increased by 20 beats per minute and this did not differ between professionals and amateurs. It was also possible to follow HRV. As I mentioned above, HRV mirrors the balance between the sympathetic and the parasympathetic.

An example illustrating one of the reasons why heart rate varies is that the heart rate increases when we inhale air, and when the air is subsequently exhaled heart rate decreases. This makes sense physiologically because when oxygenated air enters the lungs it is useful to have a large volume of blood pumped into them. On the other hand, a slower heart rhythm during exhalation allows the heart to "rest" for a short period. The professional singer who has learnt a good breathing technique adapted to singing may be more able than others to take a deep breath before the singing phrase and perhaps also utilise this kind of heart rate variability which is labelled respiratory sinus arrhythmia (RSA).

Heart rate variability is not due only to breathing. The PSS has rhythmic oscillations in its activity and so does the SS, but the frequencies of these variations are not the same and they are not the same as the breathing cycle either. Every time the PSS activity peaks, the heart rate decreases and correspondingly the heart rate increases when the SS activity peaks. The result is a complicated heart rate variability pattern with several components that can be disentangled by computer programmes. This means that within a given time interval, it is possible to assess the activity of the PSS and the SS, respectively. When we breathe normally, the heart rate variability components in this complicated web of variations can be divided into HFP (high-frequency power; 0.15–0.5 Hz corresponding to 9–30 cycles per minute), LFP (low-frequency power; 0.04–0.15 Hz corresponding to 2.4–9 cycles per minute) and VLFP (very low-frequency power; below 0.04 Hz corresponding to less than 2.4 cycles per minute). HFP is determined almost exclusively by the PSS and by breathing (which is in itself a stimulus to the parasympathetic activity). A mixture of sympathetic and parasympathetic activity is believed to determine the LFP. The VLFP, finally, is again determined by the PSS. For most people, the breathing rate is 12–18 breaths per minute when we are awake and when there is no psychological or physical exertion. During solo singing, it should be observed that a lower breathing rate than 9 cycles per minute is sometimes demanded since phrases could occasionally last for more than 7 s (corresponding to 8.6 breaths per minute or slower). This means that some of the breathing-related HRV during singing is moved from the HFP to the LFP spectrum. In addition, the difference in pressure regulation during the breathing process is different in singing than in normal breathing, and therefore, the thumb rules applied in HRV research may not always apply to singing. This may explain why LFP seems to be a more important component than HFP in some studies of singing.

The general rule for HRV is that a healthy and non-stressed individual has higher heart rate variability than a sick, depressed or exhausted subject. There is only a small variation in heart rate in an individual with deep depression or burnout. Patients who have suffered a myocardial infarction have a poor prognosis if their HRV is low. (For a more detailed description of HRV, see Porges 2007). This seems to follow a general biological rule stating that we manage our lives more effectively if we have biological flexibility. High HRV indicates that we feel well and that we are commanding our life situation in a good way. An important condition for making such conclusions from recordings, however, is that the recordings are technically good and that it is possible to distinguish abnormal heart beats and artefacts from normal heart beats. For subjects with heart disease, this may not always be possible, for instance. HRV analysis requires expert knowledge.

What happens to HRV during singing? As mentioned previously, it is likely that the breathing-related heart rate variability is important. The professional singer who is able to take a deep breath using his or her diaphragm effectively (which may result in a particularly strong parasympathetic stimulus) may also be more able than others to oxygenate blood during inhalation and allow the heart to rest during exhalation. This may result in improved ability to save energy and to keep long phrases during singing. There is evidence from our own research supporting this view.

The ECG recordings during the singing lesson in the study of amateurs and professionals (Grape 2003) showed that the HRV increased more in professionals than in amateurs when they were singing a song. This was particularly evident and statistically significant for LFP. At the same time, the professionals had an increased ratio between LFP and HFP. This is assumed to mirror a more pronounced activation of the SS. Accordingly, the professionals had a greater skill in handling the collaboration between breathing and circulation than the amateurs, but they also showed more evidence of a biological stress reaction that is consistent with the discussion above—for them the singing lesson was not for joy only. An interesting observation was that the mean heart rate during 5-min periods did not differ between the two groups—the differences were observed only when the more sophisticated measures of heart rate variability were analysed.

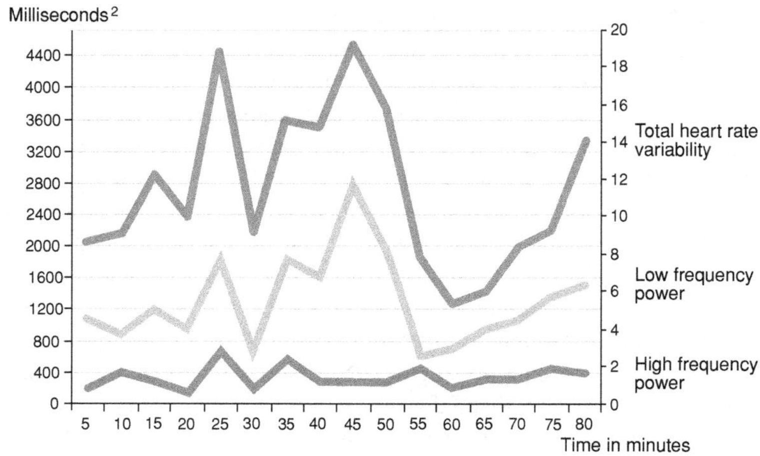

Fig. 7.1 Heart rate variability during a singing lesson in a professional singer. Minute for minute. The singing lesson lasts from the 5th to the 50th minute and is followed by resting in silence

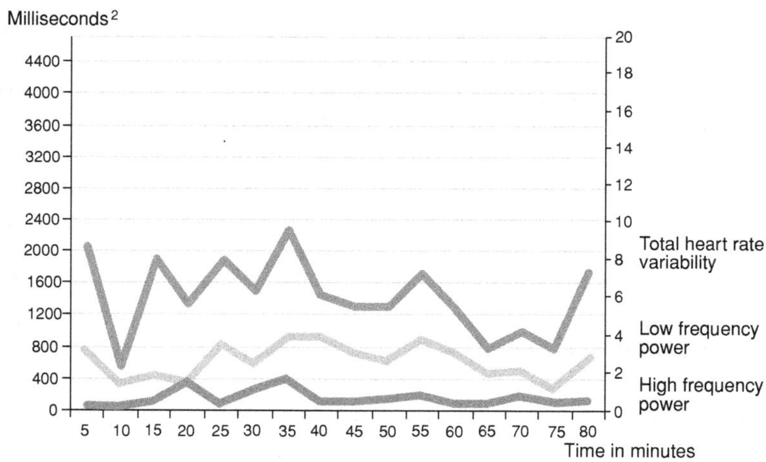

Fig. 7.2 Heart rate variability during a singing lesson in an amateur singer. Minute for minute. The singing lesson lasts from the 5th to the 50th minute and is followed by resting in silence

Figure 7.1 shows different aspects of heart rate variability during the singing lesson in a professional, and Fig. 7.2 shows corresponding data from an amateur singer. These two singers are typical of their respective groups. The figures show what happens during consecutive 5-min periods. The ECG equipment is applied to the left, and then, there is a quiet 10-min period corresponding to two 5-min periods. Thereafter, the singing lesson lasts between the 10th and the 55th minute. It starts with breathing exercises. It then continues with exercises aiming at

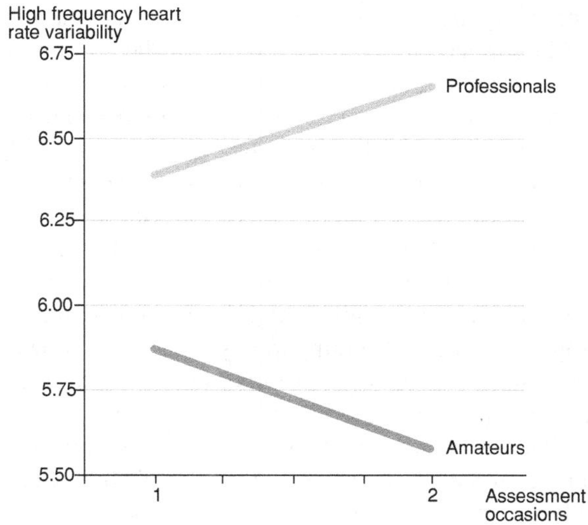

Fig. 7.3 High-frequency power variation in heart rate variability. Two assessment occasions, before start and during final singing at the end of the lesson. Natural logarithm of high-frequency-variation component of heart rate variability squared

improvement of the singer's ability to sing high and low notes, to maintain long notes and to vary strength from very soft to very strong. After this, the singer sings one or several songs. The difference in heart rate variability between the two singers is only observed during the singing of the song (35–55th minute) and not during the rest period after the lesson (55–80th minute).

Figure 7.3 shows a summary of the above, namely group means of HFP before start and during the singing of a song at the end of the lesson. The measure is expressed as the natural logarithm of milliseconds squared, which is one way of describing the "area" corresponding to the intensity of a particular part of HRV (HFP, LFP or VLFP) during this period. It is clear from the figure that the professional group increases the intensity of HFP during singing, whereas the amateur group does the opposite. These differences are statistically significant.

Hormones and Immune System

Before and after the singing lesson, venous blood was drawn for the analysis of hormonal changes after the singing lesson (Grape et al. 2003). An important observation was that the blood plasma concentration of oxytocin increased significantly both in amateurs and professionals. The oxytocin concentration increases in many situations for example during massage. Oxytocin also starts the contractions of the uterus when a child is to be born. Accordingly, the effect of singing is not a specific one. Animal experiments have shown (see Uvnäs Moberg 1997) that oxytocin stimulates learning and that it is of importance for the attachment between infant and mother. Theories have also been developed regarding the "oxytocinergic" system in the brain. It has been hypothesised to be of importance to the development of the parasympathetic nervous system. This may mean that children growing up in dangerous stressful situations develop a good ability to identify and deal with stress but not such a good ability to activate oxytocin which stands for calmness and safety. Oxytocin may, because of its role in learning, stimulate curiosity. And animal research (Grippo et al. 2012) has shown that oxytocin injections during a period of isolation may protect the body from adverse effects of a stressful situation. In other words, oxytocin seems to have a protective role in relation to adverse effects of negative stress reactions. Most of this is highly speculative and exactly how we can link massage, learning and singing to oxytocin is not known. It is likely that lullabies and caressing may be of great importance to brain functions in the small child, and some of this may be mediated by oxytocin.

The oxytocin effect of the singing lesson was the same in amateurs and professionals. There were, however, differences in other biological systems. The most striking difference was observed for TNF alpha. This is a pro-inflammatory cytokine—a group of immune-chemical agents in the body stimulating inflammatory reactions that are part of the defence in stress situations. TNF alpha increases fatigue. A speculative interpretation of this is that the immune system wants to give a chemical signal to the brain that there is need for a rest! The plasma concentration of TNF alpha increased significantly in the professional singers but not at all in the amateurs. Perhaps, this means that the stress reaction in the professional singers was also activating the immune system.

How can we interpret the "good" performance of the HRV during singing alone, with the biological stress reaction in the sympathetic nervous system and in the pro-inflammatory immune system in the professional singers, while the amateur singers perform more poorly with regard to HRV while they have no stress reaction? The explanation may be that the professionals are more skilful but also more engaged in their task and therefore also more stressed in this particular situation. Stress is here defined as bodily arousal in a situation that requires excessive energy. The professionals have learnt how to activate the parasympathetic response, with large variations in heart rate, while they have a high sympathetic arousal—the two opposing systems are activated at the same time! This is a relatively unexplored research field so we have no clear answers.

A German study (Kreutz et al. 2004) has examined changes in the immune system in choir singers from before to after a choir rehearsal. The concentration of plasma immunoglobulin A increased significantly after the choir rehearsal, and no such effect was observed after listening to the same music. Accordingly, the immune system is engaged while we sing. This finding is interpreted as positive since immunoglobulin A contributes to the defence against infections. We do not know how long lasting such effects are and whether a repeated activation of this part of the immune system once a week has a beneficial effect on health.

Heart Rate: Physical Work

How much elevation of heart rate does singing give rise to? The small study of the singing lesson shows that the effects on average heart rate per 5-min period are relatively small. The maximal heart rate was between 105 and 115 beats per minute, and the effect was the same for amateurs and professionals. A real audience, however, does make considerable difference with much more pronounced heart rate elevation. Many experience nervousness when they are going to perform, singing in front of an audience. This has frequently been labelled stage fright, which is an adequate description of the feeling. Another way of describing it is to say that the performer wants the audience to love the song just as much as the singer does—he or she wants to transmit an emotional message. This causes considerable arousal. However, if the singer forgets himself/herself and devotes all effort to the message in the song, the audience gets engaged and a wordless communication arises. Such a state is labelled flow. It is characterised by a high level of arousal, a feeling that the performer is successfully managing something that is difficult and finally an elated emotion (Ullén et al. 2010). Its physiological correlates will be described below. Before this theme is discussed more in detail, I shall illustrate with a couple of examples how the heart rate itself is affected. Regardless of the emotional correlates of the performance, there is an elevation of heart rate.

Two examples from my own singing of two different songs that I have performed without and with audience will serve as illustrations. These songs were performed with ECG "online" recording in front of an audience on several occasions. I have also performed them in the same way without audience. The first song (PB, music see Fig. 7.4, page 81 in Swedish version) "Sång efter skördeanden" (Song after harvest) is well known in Sweden. It is by composer Peterson Berger (1867–1942) with autobiographic lyrics by Karlfeldt (1864–1931). Range E to a flat—normal for a tenor. It is a proud forceful waltz with some high notes. The phrases do not exceed 7 s. The second song (R, music see Fig. 7.5) "Den enda stunden" (The only moment) is also well known in the Swedish setting. The music is by Rangström (1884–1947) and the lyrics by Runeberg (1804–1877). Range E to e. The phrases do not exceed 7 s. This is a soft impressionistic song about two individuals who meet and do not take the opportunity of talking to one another although for a moment they are tempted to do so.

The heart rate variations beat for beat for the first (PB) song are presented in Fig. 7.4 and the corresponding data for the second song (R) in Fig. 7.5. The recordings contain some artefacts caused by contractions in skeletal muscles. One has to disregard those (vertical lines).

My heart rate at rest is 50 beats per minute. When I sing the more strenuous song without audience, my heart rate peaks at 90 beats per minute in the more physically demanding parts. When I sing this song to an audience, my heart rate peaks at 130–140 beats per minute (always when I sing the highest notes, a flat and g). The other softer song is associated with less elevation of heart rate with maximum 70 without and 90 with an audience. A high heart rate corresponds to a high degree of physical

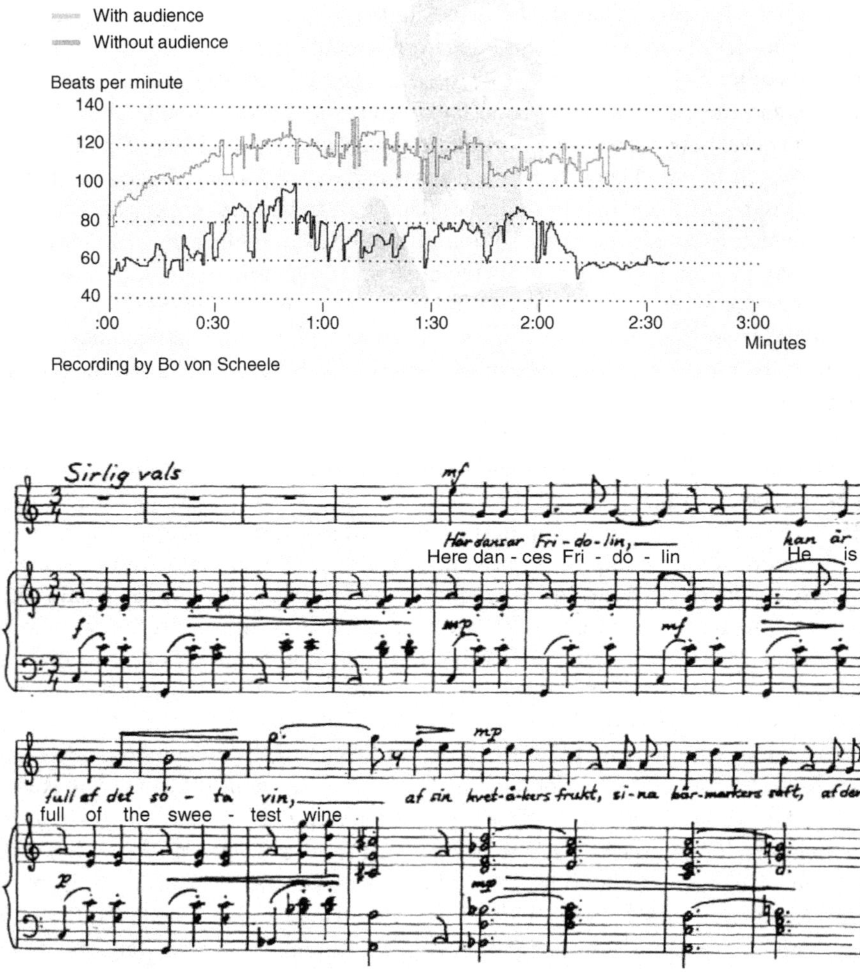

Fig. 7.4 Heart rate variations during singing. The author sings *Sång efter skördeanden* (Song after harvest) by Peterson-Berger (music) and Karlfeldt (words): "Here dances Fridolin, he is full of the sweetest wine…"

engagement. If we compare this to a situation in the training gym, we may notice that a standardised effort at the treadmill starts to get strenuous approximately at 140 beats per minute. Accordingly, some parts of the singing, at least when it is performed in front of an audience, correspond to a considerable physical effort. It is well known to all singers that the body may get warm and even sweating after long-lasting singing. Hard physical work entails excessive calorie production.

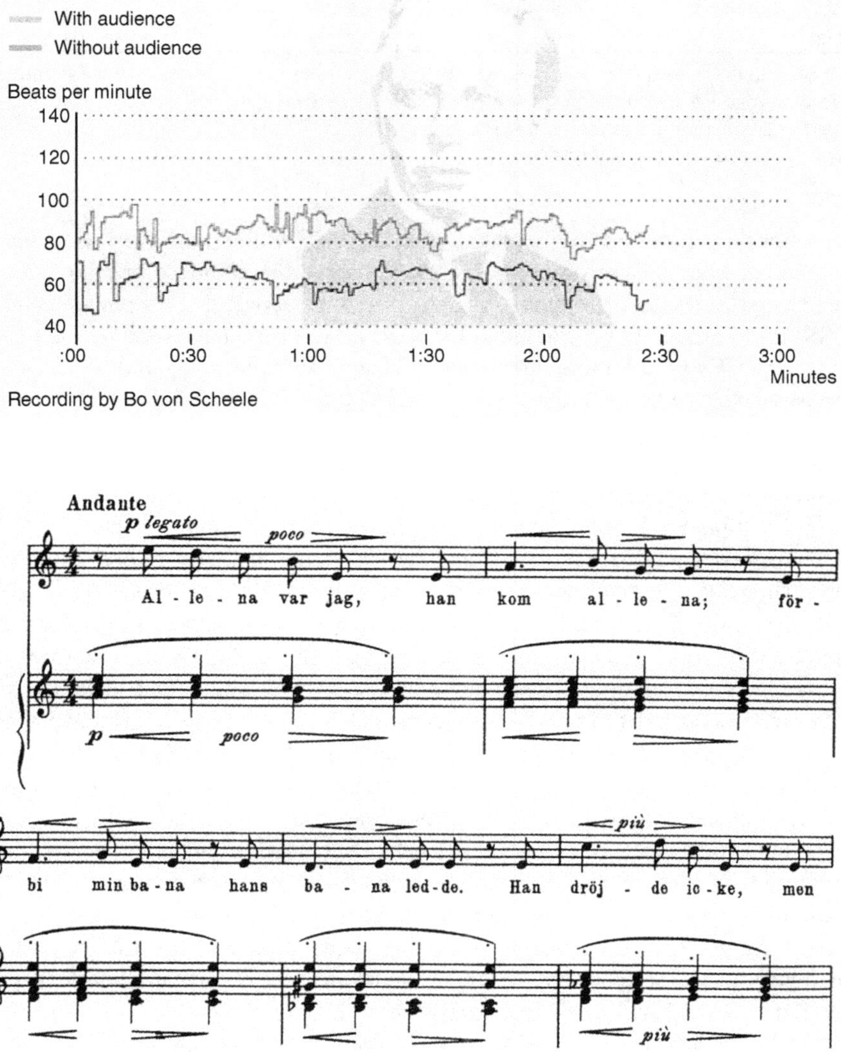

Fig. 7.5 Heart rate variations during singing. The author sings *Den enda stunden* (The unique moment) by Rangström (music) and Runeberg: "I wandered lonely…"

The heart rate recordings of myself also show that HRV is affected differently by the different situations. Disregarding the vertical lines caused by muscular artefacts, it is clear that the heart rate variability is much smaller when I sing the more

Table 7.2 Mean LFP from HRV (natural logarithm of ms squared for low-frequency power) during ten pairs of music performances (professional flute players and singers)—"strenuous" and "easy" piece with and without audience

Ln LFP on average during			
Easy piece		Strenuous piece	
Without audience	With audience	Without audience	With audience
2,981	735	2,208	493

Those who did not experience nervousness before had during the performance of the strenuous piece average 1,620 during concert while those who reported nervousness before concert had average 206 during the corresponding situation
Source Harmat and Theorell (2010)

strenuous song with an audience than when I do it without an audience. The difference in HRV is less obvious when we observe the audience and no audience recordings of the less strenuous song. As discussed above, the sympathetic and the PSSs may sometimes be aroused at the same time. There are several online recordings when I sing the more strenuous (PB) song in front of an audience. On one occasion, the audience looked very friendly and this affected my own feeling. I felt like dancing a waltz. The recordings from that singing episode show the same heart rate averages but a higher HRV—as if the parasympathetic and SSs were concomitantly activated.

So far I have only discussed one case. In one study (Harmat and Theorell 2010), we have performed continuous ECG recordings during ten pairs of performances of one "strenuous" (long phrases, strong force, high notes, etc.) and one "easy" piece, with and without an audience. The musicians were professional singers and flute players (flute playing is very similar to singing). The results seem to illustrate several of the points that I have described in the case study. Tables 7.1 and 7.2 show the group results for heart rate and for one aspect of HRV (LFP, low-frequency power).

Both the degree of difficulty and the audience have an effect on the average heart rate, but it is clear that the audience effect is stronger (+22 beats per minute in the easy and +27 beats per minute in the strenuous piece) than the effect of the strenuous versus easy piece (+4 beats per minute without audience and +9 beats per minute with audience). A parallel phenomenon is observed for the heart rate variability, with a very strong effect of the audience and a small effect of the easy versus strenuous piece. Another interesting observation was that the effect of the audience during performance of the strenuous piece was particularly strong when the performer felt nervous before the concert (average 206 for the nervous versus 1,620 in the non-nervous). HRV showed a much stronger correlation with nervousness than did heart rate. This is in line with the case observations on myself discussed above.

In this case, LFP was the component of HRV that discriminated the most clearly. This may be due to the fact that we recorded professional performances and some of the musical phrases were long. According to the discussion above, long phrases exceeding 7 s could cause drifting of heart rate variability from the high-frequency to the low-frequency domain. In addition, as I pointed out

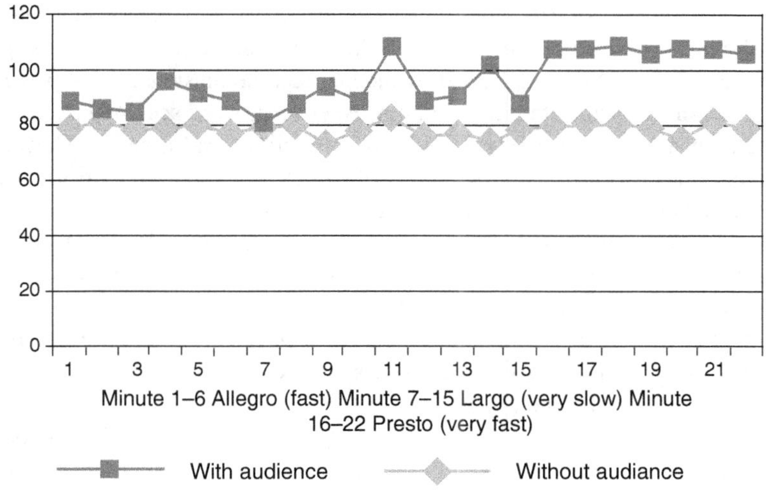

Fig. 7.6 Mean heart rate minute after minute in professional pianist who is playing the Ghost Trio for piano, violin and cello by Beethoven with/without audience

previously, a successful concert performance by a professional may be characterised by a mixture of parasympathetic and sympathetic arousal. The high skill level makes it possible for the professional to focus on the emotional message and the totality of the performance despite a high arousal level—since little conscious attention has to be paid to the technical details of the performance.

From these descriptions, it may be possible to identify a few factors that may be of importance to the biological effects of singing:

1. The singer's skill
2. The human surrounding, if there is an audience and how the audience behaves (supportive or critical)
3. The technical demands in the song (force, pitch, difficult or simple intervals, complicated or simple rhythms, length of phrases)
4. The emotional engagement (flow or negative feelings)

As we have seen, breathing is of such great importance to singing that it would be interesting to compare with musical performance that is not so intimately related to the breathing cycle. In an unpublished case study, we were able to follow the ECG recordings of a professional pianist when he performed a difficult piece of chamber music, the "ghost trio" by Ludvig van Beethoven both without and with an audience. The average heart rate minute after minute is displayed in Fig. 7.6. The blue curve shows the heart rate without audience. It is stable and always around 80 beats per minute. During concert, however, there is more minute-to-minute variation with a total mean of 95 beats per minute. During the most difficult last movement, presto, the heart rate is between 105 and 108 beats per minute. Accordingly, the heart rate difference between the concert and the audience-free situation is of the same order of magnitude as the corresponding heart rate difference for singers and flute players. It should be pointed out that—as with the singers and flute players—the performance during concert is complicated by the fact that the musician is not performing alone. The singers and flute players in our experiment were accompanied by piano and the pianist even had two co-musicians—a violinist and a cellist. During concert when tension rises, a high tempo is often selected (perhaps mirroring a high heart rate!). This is exactly what happened in the piano example. The tempo in the presto movement became very fast, and hence, the technical difficulties were unusually pronounced. In conclusion, the audience effect on heart rate may be approximately the same for pianists as it is for singers and flute players. Piano teachers have started thinking along these lines and instruct their pupils about breathing techniques in order to improve playing technique—despite the lack of immediate association between breathing and piano playing.

A more detailed study of the flow state (de Manzano et al. 2010) found in pianists has been published. Twenty-one professional solo pianists participated. They were asked to play in the laboratory a difficult self-selected piece that they liked. After each performance, they were asked with the use of a standardised questionnaire to rate the degree of flow that they had experienced. The performances were ranked with regard to flow, and online physiological recordings were analysed in relation to the flow experience. The flow experience was characterised by a high heart rate, relaxed chewing muscles and deep breathing. This could be interpreted as evidence of concomitant sympathetic and parasympathetic arousal. The theory of "effortless attention" (=flow) in relation to physiology has been discussed by Ullén et al. (2010). So far, research has only shown that the physiological state accompanying the state of flow differs from the physiology of destructive "stress" (attention with effort) in the sense that the regulation of physiological functions is more optimal during flow.

In the next chapter, I shall discuss choir singing. To sing in a group is something more than to sing alone!

References

De Manzano, Ö., Harmat, L., Theorell, T., & Ullén, F. (2010). The pathophysiology of flow during piano playing. *Emotion, 10*(3), 301–311.

Grape, C., Sandgren, M., Hansson, L.-O., Ericson, M., & Theorell, T. (2003). Does singing promote well-being? An empirical study of professional and amateur singers during a singing lesson. *Integrative Physiological and Behavioural Science, 38*, 65–74.

Grippo, A. J., Pournajafi-Nazarloo, H., Sanzenbacher, L., Trahanas, D. M., McNeal, N., Clarke, D. A., et al. (2012). Peripheral oxytocin administration buffers autonomic but not behavioral responses to environmental stressors in isolated prairie voles. *Stress, 15*(2), 149–161. doi:10.3109/10253890.2011.605486. Epub 19 Aug 2011.

Harmat, L., & Theorell, T. (2010). Heart rate variability during singing and flute playing. *Music and Medicine, 2*, 10–17.

Kleber, B., Veit, R., Birbaumer, N., Gruzelier, L., & Lotze, M. (2010). The brain of opera singers: experience-dependent changes in functional activation. *Cerebral Cortex, 20*, 1144–1152.

Kreutz, G., Bongard, S., Rohrmann, S., Hodapp, V., & Grebe, D. (2004). Effects of choir singing or listening on secretory immunoglobulin A, cortisol, and emotional state. *Journal of Behavioral Medicine, 27*(6), 623–635.

Porges, S. W. (2007). The polyvagal perspective. *Biological Psychology, 74*(2), 116–143.

Sandgren, M., & Borg, E. (2009). Immediate effects of choral singing on emotional states: Differences in groups with lower and higher health status. *Opublicerat manuskript.*

Sundberg, J. (1989). *The science of the singing voice.* DeKalb :Northern Illinois University Press.

Ullén, F., de Manzano, Ö., Harmat, L., & Theorell, T. (2010). The physiology of effortless attention: Correlates of state flow and flow proneness. In: B. Bruya (Ed.), *Effortless attention. A new perspective in the cognitive science of attention and action* (pp. 205–217). Cambridge: The MIT Press.

Uvnäs Moberg, K. (1997). Oxytocin linked antistress effects—The relaxation and growth response. *Acta physiologica scandinavica, 161*(suppl 640), 38–42.

Wilson, S. J., Abbott, D. F., Lusher, D., Gentle, E. C., & Jackson, G. D. (2010). Finding your voice: A singing lesson from functional imaging. *Human Brain Mapping, 32*(12), 2115–2130. doi: 10.1002/hbm.21173 (epub 2010 Dec 15).

Chapter 8
Singing Together

Statistical data on choir singing in the Swedish population has been produced since the early 1980s by the National Survey of Living Conditions ("Undersökningen om Levnadsförhållanden", ULF). This study is based upon face-to-face interviews with large samples of randomly selected men and women. Among many things, it has comprised questions about cultural activities. This allows us to follow the development from 1982 to 2006 (for a brief summary, see Theorell and Kreutz 2012). During the first years (1982–1991), 3.5 % of all Swedes in the ages 16–84 were singing in a choir at least once a week. This percentage increased to 3.7–3.8 % in the years 1998–2006. However, most of this small increase was due to the fact that older people started singing in a choir more frequently. In the oldest category, the percentage singing in a choir once a week was only 1.4 % in 1982–1983, whereas in 2006, it was 4.6 %. In the youngest category (16–19 years), there was no change (9.1–7.0 % in 1982–1983 and 1990–1991 and 7.4 % in 1998–1999 and 8.3 % in 2006). If we extend the choir singing to "singing at least once last year in a choir", the numbers were higher, again with a small continuous increase for the whole period—from 5.3 % in 1982–1983 to 5.9 % in 2006. In all ages, we can see that choir singing is more popular among women than among men. For instrument playing, the gender difference is in the opposite direction, with men playing instruments more frequently than women. There is also a social gradient, with highly educated men and women more frequently performing music than less educated.

There is no strictly comparable data set in any other country. However, in a report from the United States (The Chorus Impact Study 2009) based upon households rather than individuals, it was reported that in 18.1 % of households in the USA, at least one adult member participates in a choir. This indicates that there has been an increasing interest in choir singing from 2003 in the USA (when the corresponding percentage of households was 15.6 %). If children are included, the corresponding number in 2009 was 22.9 % of the households. However, the authors in this report note that there has been a slight decrease in choir singing among children.

T. Theorell, *Psychological Health Effects of Musical Experiences*,
SpringerBriefs in Psychology, DOI: 10.1007/978-94-017-8920-2_8,

In summary, choir singing is a popular leisure time activity. There are indications that participation in a choir increases among elderly and decreases slightly among children and teenagers.

Many people report increased well-being when they sing regularly in a choir. Several studies have been published in which choir members have been interviewed regarding their experiences. For example, Clift and Hancox (2001) interviewed elderly choir singers while Sandgren and Borg (2009) interviewed mixed age adult choir singers of varying degrees of expertise, ranging from professionals to less advanced amateurs, all singing classical music. In Lindström's study (2006), the emphasis was on choir singing in types of choirs that have not existed before, such as rehabilitation choirs, health choirs, job choirs, etc. An increasingly popular kind of choir is the one for those who have never sung before—"beginner's choirs". These choirs are often large, sometimes including several hundred people. I know personally several men and women who have started singing in such a choir in their middle or old age who report that this has been dramatically uplifting to the extent that it has "positively changed their lives".

As a general rule, a high level of education increases the likelihood of participation in cultural activities. There are interesting exceptions to this rule, however. This was for example the case in a newly published Norwegian study (Vaag et al. 2012). In this study, all staffs in two county hospitals were offered the opportunity to participate in joint rock singing—a kind of well-being choir at work. After rehearsals, the participants gave a concert. A sum of 1431 employees completed a survey questionnaire after the concert (57 % of singers plus employees in the audience responded to the questionnaire). Thirty per cent of those who responded had actually participated in the singing. Low participation in the choir singing activity was found among men (compared to women), employees above 62 and below 38 years of age (compared to those between 38 and 62 years of age), part-time employees (compared to full-time working), university educated workers (compared to those with lower education) and health care workers (compared to other employees). The likelihood of participation is determined by a number of factors. The kind of music activity is of course a factor of decisive importance, and it interacts with age, gender, ethnic group and type of employment. In the Norwegian job, example rock music singing appealed particularly to middle-aged women without higher education. Classical music, gospel and folk music may appeal to other groups.

In the interviews with elderly people singing in a choir, spontaneous statements of relevance to wellbeing have been systematically grouped (Clift and Hancox 2001). The most common kinds of well-being statements relate to the joy and togetherness that choir singers experience. This is a powerful amplifier of social support and is of importance to health because these people feel a strengthened motivation to adopt a healthy lifestyle. The singing brings meaning to their lives. In many of these choral groups organised for the elderly, we are frequently talking about unison song without chords. Elite goals are unimportant. On the other hand, it is important not to trivialise the choice of music or to underestimate the ability of the participants. To find a reasonable goal that is accepted by the majority is a challenge for the leader. The effect on cohesiveness with the group may be the most important one, and it will be discussed more in detail below. The choice of music, the leader's attitude to the participants' singing ability and socio-economic conditions is substantial. Negative associations with choir singing have also been described in written responses to open-ended questions in a large-scale survey with 3,145 subjects (Kreutz and Brünger 2012). Social problems as well as conflicting aesthetic goals dominate in such negative statements.

It should be remembered that statements from choir singers that they feel healthier than people in general do not prove that choir singing caused good health. Those who develop certain kinds of illnesses are likely to stop participating in choir singing. Accordingly, some of this association could be due to reversed causality—healthy people are more likely to sing in a choir! Therefore, studies are needed which are based upon subjects who start singing in a choir and are followed for longer periods of time, not only when they sing. A wide range of health parameters could be studied.

Health effects of choir singing include such effects that were discussed in the previous chapter about individual singing:

Aesthetic and emotional surprises resulting in changed life goals and coping patterns

Physical training

Improved coordination between breathing and circulation

Balance between the sympathetic and parasympathetic systems

Hormonal changes (oxytocin, beta-endorphin for example)

But in choir singing, there is also the cohesiveness effect. Perhaps we are even genetically programmed to feel strong togetherness when we make sounds together. Throughout mankind's history, human beings have performed dance and music in their religious rituals. Perhaps the overriding goal of this has been to strengthen cohesiveness in order to make group members collaborate effectively. Individuals who have not been able to participate in such activities may have had a smaller chance of survival than others. Could it even be that after tens of thousands of years this has resulted in genetic selection of subjects with ability to participate in music and dance? I have introduced this kind of reasoning earlier in this book. It may explain why tone deafness is very uncommon in the general population.

A phenomenon that has been examined in recent studies is the extent to which breathing and heart are coordinated during choir singing. A recently published study (Vickhoff et al. 2013) showed that a small group of choir singers who were singing a slow relaxed unison song coordinated their breathing. This may contribute to the feeling of togetherness. On the other hand, when words are added and the music becomes more complex (different parts; soprano, alto, tenor and bass) breathing becomes less coordinated (Olsson et al. 2013).

Challenges may be important for health effects. A choir may face a difficult piece and may initially doubt its ability to perform it (perhaps at a concert!). If it succeeds well, the feeling of achievement may be a strong health promotion factor in itself. If it fails, there may be opposite effects.

In an experiment, we examined whether choir singing once a week during a whole year for beginners had the same effect as a comparison programme, in which participants received short lectures and discussed their contents. The time allotted to the lectures and the singing was the same in the two groups during the study period. Participants were recruited among patients with irritable bowel syndrome (IBS). None of them had been singing in a choir, but wanted to start doing so. For participation in the study, they had to accept that they would be allocated randomly to one of the two groups. IBS symptoms (oscillation between constipation and diarrhoea, flatulence and pain) are partly determined by psychological reactions to stress and partly by a number of physical factors such as aberrations in meal rhythm and diet. IBS is a common illness (in a study of German students 18 %, Gulewitsch et al. 2011) and may periodically be incapacitating although it is not life threatening. IBS patients have been described in the literature as bodily sensitive to external stimuli and stress. Since participants in both groups were involved in group activities, cohesiveness effects could have been obtained in both, and if the choir group would turn out to differ from the other group, the difference would likely be due to the group singing as such.

Several factors were assessed in the two IBS groups, before starting, as well as after 6, 9 and 12 months. First, I would like to report findings (Grape et al. 2010) on a factor that is of importance because it reflects the body's regenerative activity, which was discussed in the previous chapter on stress. Regeneration is important because there is a constant breakdown of cells in all tissues in the body—in the skin, the immune system, the mucosa, the muscles, the connective tissue, the bones and the cells supporting the brain cells (Horvitz 2003). If the body downplays (which it tends to do during periods of excessive negative stress) this supportive activity, the body suffers and illness will arise sooner or later. In order to give the reader a concrete idea of this, it has been calculated that on average, we need to replace 1.5 kg of cells every day. The half-life of cells differs across different organ systems. There is a very slow turnover of skeletal cells (years) and a rapid destruction of white blood cells (days), for example. One important theory regarding music's possible health promoting effect is that it may stimulate regenerative activity, just like regular, wise physical exercise may do.

A regenerative hormone that is relatively easy to assess is testosterone. This is one of the male sex hormones (anabolic steroids) that constitute a problem in sports. We associate them with illegal administration of high dosages. Both men and women have testosterone. Men have 10–20 times more testosterone in blood than women but most of the excess testosterone in men is tied to globulins and not immediately accessible. "Free" testosterone on the other hand is excreted into saliva, where the levels are more similar in men and women (men have approximately 50–100 % higher concentration in saliva than women). In addition, the concentration of testosterone in saliva is regulated physiologically in such a way that when the individual feels fine and has a good mental state, the saliva testosterone concentration increases (mirroring increasing regeneration) and vice versa, both in men and women.

In the study of choir singing and IBS, the participants were asked to collect saliva on six occasions during an assessment day—when they woke up, half an hour after waking up, at lunch, before the activity (choir or group talk), after the activity and finally before going to bed. Means were calculated from those six assessments. This testosterone mean showed a 60 % increase during the first 6 months of choir singing group, whereas no such change was observed in the talk group. When the development was analysed, the difference between the groups was shown to have decreased from 6 to 9 months and then further from 9 to 12 months after the start. Visual analogue scales were used for the IBS participants in both groups who were asked to rate the degree of tiredness/vitality that they felt before and after choir/talk. These assessments showed that after 4 months, there was no vitality effect in the talk group but a pronounced and highly significant such effect after the choir activity.

In summary, the "vitality" effect that has been so frequently reported after choir rehearsals in other studies was obvious 4 months after these beginners had started choral singing. The testosterone effect that was measured after 6 months is consistent with this and may mirror an increased regeneration activity in the participants. However, the effect did not last until the end of the study year. We can only speculate about reasons for this—perhaps the choir group was not as stimulating in the end as it was in the beginning. We have to know more about how to make the choir effect last longer.

Samples of venous blood were also collected from the IBS participants before and after the study year (Grape et al. 2008) for the assessment of fibrinogen. Fibrinogen mirrors the activity in the pro-inflammatory part of the immune system; during periods of arousal the concentration of it in blood plasma increases and vice versa. Broadly speaking, it can be used as an index of catabolism, using the terminology that was introduced in the chapter about stress. High levels of plasma fibrinogen are associated with increased risk of developing cardiovascular disease. There was a significant difference between the groups with regard to fibrinogen, lasting through the whole study year: After half a year, the concentration had decreased in the choir group while it had increased in the talk group. Twelve months after starting, the choir group still had a significant advantage over the talk group although the difference had decreased. Similarly, after 12 months, a hormone regulating the bowel movements and therefore of direct significance for the IBS itself, motilin, showed a slight decrease in the choir group and a slight increase in the talk group, resulting in an almost significant difference between the groups. An exact parallel was observed during the study year with regard to pain related to IBS; a slight decrease in the choir group and a slight increase in the talk group, resulting in an almost significant difference between the groups.

The IBS choir experiment that I have described in detail was not a perfect one. In both study groups, there was a drop out—only 50 % in both groups participated until the end of the study year. The final number of participants after 12 months was relatively small, 13 in the choir group and 14 in the other group. Even at the beginning, our participants were not representative of the normal population—all of them had IBS, all wanted to start singing in a choir, and all had accepted the special study conditions including random allocation. It could perhaps be argued that the activity in the comparison group may have been a disappointment for those participants. This was not the case! They were quite satisfied with the lectures and group discussions that they had during the study year. We need more studies of this kind. However, the tentative findings point in the direction that I outlined in the stress chapter—choir singing once a week may not only have temporary effects during and immediately after the choir activity. Effects in the direction of reduced catabolism (reduced fibrinogen mirroring "negative stress") and improved anabolism (increased testosterone mirroring improved resistance against stress) may take place. In addition, the design makes it likely that no group activity is likely to equal the effect of regular group singing.

The type of study that the IBS study represents does not give us any clue as to what it is in choir singing that may have positive health effects. Is it the training of the improved collaboration between lungs and heart? Is it the aesthetic experience that starts a new orientation in life? What is the significance of the concerted bodily movements that the members are making during singing? A study of the neurohormonal effects of tango dancing (Quiroga et al. 2009) has shown that the close presence of a partner stimulates the saliva secretion of testosterone, a finding quite in line with our finding on testosterone. At any rate, the results of our study indicate that group singing may add something important psychologically and biologically to the general group effect of people meeting once a week to talk.

The evidence in the scientific literature on possible positive health effects of choir singing hitherto is actually scant. In a review, Clift (2012) has recently concluded that the support from experimental studies of health effects of choral singing is modest. (See also Clift et al. 2010). Most of the evidence for a health effect is indirect. The findings in Hyyppä's (2007) research (see above) indicate that choir singing may be an important ingredient in the social capital that seems to explain the longevity of Swedish-speaking East Bothnians in Finland. Choir singing of a specific kind in a given social context may contribute to longevity.

Another study (Cohen 2009), which supports that regular choir singing may have real health effects is the study performed on elderly institutionalised subjects in Washington DC. All potential participants wanted to start singing in a choir. Two comparable groups were established. Half of them started singing in a choir once a week for 2 years, while the other half had to wait for 2 years. Standardised questionnaires were used before, after one year and after 2 years for the assessment of health. The findings showed that the choir singing subjects were favoured with regard to health development.

The ability of music to make "short cuts" to the emotional brain and to trigger unexpected psychological processes has been discussed above. This, in combination with a strong social experience arising in group singing, may explain why it is possible to rapidly establish a vitalising effect, psychologically and biologically, when a choral group is established. As I have pointed out, there are also direct physical effects of training large muscle groups (diaphragm and breathing muscles), approximately as is done in regular physical exercise, and of coordinating breathing and circulation (see the discussion regarding the effects of professional singing education).

Inexperienced singers, however, may experience fear when they are singing in a small group. This may threaten the good effects of group singing. This may be one explanation why some of the good health effects were attenuated during the latter part of the study year in the IBS study. Since there were relatively few participants in some of the rehearsals, some individuals may have felt "exposed" when singing almost solo.

Different kinds of choirs—a gospel choir, a rehabilitation choir, a choir for elderly or a beginner's choir—work in very different ways. They are also working in a way that is completely different from the way in which a professional choir is operating, for instance. In the gospel choir rhythm, religious experiences and improvisation are in focus. In the rehabilitation choir, the choir leader has the responsibility of finding out what the needs of the participants are and build the activities on those needs. Only a music therapist can do this. In the (mostly) large beginner's choirs, the participants want to have experiences on an existential level that they have not had any experiences on before. In the professional choir, all participants have to be highly educated and skilful singers with high musical commitment, and a beginner would feel very unwelcome.

The effects of singing in different kinds of choirs are very different also. In a beginner's choir, the strongest effect may have to do with strengthened assertiveness. One of the choir participants in the IBS study expressed that in the following way: "Now I can sing *Happy birthday to you* with the family without feeling ashamed!" This of course relates to the fact that many adults suffer from humiliating experiences when they were children. They may have been labelled as tone deaf or completely without musicality and now they discover that they can in fact sing. When they start training their singing voice, they frequently also improve quality of speaking, and of course speaking well clearly is a very important part of life.

A special kind of choir is the workplace choir. Its existence may stimulate cohesiveness and creativity. There are even workplaces in which recruitments are based partly on singing ability! However, such activities of course have to be voluntary. Many people hate singing, and it is of course impossible to force employees to participate in choir singing at work. There should also be awareness among enthusiastic choir singers that if only a few of the employees participate in this activity, a strong group cohesion may arise which may make other employees feel excluded. Other cultural activities could then be organised so that all employees feel culturally stimulated and are able to contribute.

For those of us who have experienced the painstaking detailed work in a choir with high musical aspirations, it is quite clear that the rehearsals are not always wonderful. They may even become boring, and we might doubt our ability to perform a difficult programme. However, when everything works and the totality (perhaps orchestra, soloists, etc.) becomes obvious, strong cohesiveness effects may arise that are closely associated with the aesthetic experiences. I have myself had very strong such experiences standing beside somebody who sings another voice in the choir while, on the other side, there is somebody who sings the same voice as I do. If the chords and the rhythm are working perfectly together, one forgets oneself, feeling that one is part of a huge organ. This basic feeling is probably very similar in different kinds of choirs. One has to go through frustration, insecurity and goal-directed training in order to be able to experience such satisfaction! This principle could also be applied to music in children's lives which is the subject of the next chapter.

References

Clift, S. M., & Hancox, G. (2001). The perceived benefits of singing: Findings from preliminary surveys of a university college choral society. *The Journal of the Royal Society for the Promotion of Health, 121*, 248–256.

Clift, S., Hancox, G., Morrison, I., Hess, B., Kreutz, G., & Stewart, D. (2010). Choral singing and psychological wellbeing: Quantitative and qualitative findings from English choirs in a cross-national survey. *Journal of Applied Arts and Health, 1*(1), 19–34. doi:10.1386/jaah.1.1.19/1.

Clift, S. M. (2012). Singing, wellbeing, and health. In R. Macdonald, G. Kreutz & L. Mitchell (Eds.), *Music, health and wellbeing* (pp. 113–124). Oxford: Oxford University Press.

Cohen, G. (2009). New theories and research findings on the positive influence of music and art on health with ageing. *Arts and Health, 1*, 48–62.

Grape, C., Theorell, T., Wikström, B. M., & Ekman, R. (2008). Choir singing and fibrinogen. VEGF, cholecystokinin and motilin in IBS patients. *Medical Hypotheses, 72*, 223–234.

Grape, C., Wikström, B.-M., Ekman, R., Hasson, D., & Theorell, T. (2010). Comparison between choir singing and group discussion in irritable bowel syndrome patients over one year: Saliva testosterone increases in new choir singers. *Psychotherapy and Psychosomatics, 79*, 196–198.

Gulewitsch, M. D., Enck, P., Hautzinger, M., & Schlarb, A. A. (2011). Irritable bowel syndrome symptoms among German students: Prevalence, characteristics and associations to somatic complaints, sleep quality of life and childhood abdominal pain. *European Journal of Gastroenterology and Hepatology, 23*, 311–316.

Horvitz HR (2003) Worms, life and death (Nobel lecture)—Review. ChemBiochem, 697–711.

Hyyppä, M. T. (2007). *Livskraft ur gemenskap (Life energy from cohesion)*. Lund: Student literature.

Kreutz, G., & Brünger, P. (2012). A shade of grey: Negative associations with amateur choral singing. *Arts and Health, 4*, 230–238.

Lindström, D. (2006). Sjung, sjung för livet! En studie av körsång som pedagogisk verksamhet och av deltagarnas upplevelse av hälsa och livskvalitet. (Sing, sing for life! A study of choral singing as pedagogical activity and of participant experiences of health and quality of life). Academic Thesis, Luleå Technical University and the College of Music in Piteå, 43 (ISSN: 1402-1757), Luleå.

Olsson, E. M. G., von Schéele, B., & Theorell, T. (2013). Heart rate variability during choral singing music and medicine. Published online 10 Jan 2013. doi:10.1177/1943862112471399.

Quiroga Murcia, C., Bongard, S., & Kreutz, G. (2009). Emotional and neurohumoral responses to dancing tango argentino. The effects of music and partner. *Music and Medicine, 1*, 14–21.

Sandgren, M., & Borg, E. (2009). Immediate effects of choral singing on emotional states: Differences in groups with lower and higher health status. *Unpublished manuscript*.

Theorell, T., & Kreutz, G. (2012). Epidemiological studies of the relationship between musical experiences and public health. In R. MacDonald, G. Kreutz & L. Mitchell (Eds.), *Music, health, and wellbeing* (pp. 424–435). Oxford: Oxford University Press.

Vaag, J., Saksvik, P. Ö., Theorell, T., Skillingstad, T., & Bjerkeset, O. (2012). Sound of well-being—Choir singing as an intervention to improve well-being among employees in two Norwegian county hospitals. *Arts and Health*,. doi:10.1080/17533015.2012.727838.

Vickhoff, B., Malmgren, H., Åström, R., Nyberg, G., Engvall, M., Snygg, J., et al. (2013). Music structure determines heart rate variability of singers. *Frontiers in psychology, 4*, 334. doi:10.3389/fpsyg.2013.00334.

Chapter 9
Growing up with Music

Children who grow up with music, do they get any advantages of this—apart from having musical experiences? Since music is so important in communication and since we may even be genetically predisposed with a sense of rhythm and music may even be "prepared", it may be particularly important to have musical input during childhood. The development of emotional competence may to a great extent be influenced by music. Accordingly, do children who are stimulated by an abundance of musical experiences become emotionally more competent as adults than others? A parallel discussion relates to cognitive development. There is research indicating that the cognitive development may also be stimulated by early music training. If it is true that music stimulates both emotional and cognitive skills, a lot of musical training would be very important to give all children.

In psychosomatic medicine, the concept *alexithymia* is important. This means ability to differentiate feelings. A person who has a good ability to identify, describe, differentiate and deal with different emotions has a great advantage in life. Those who lack this ability suffer from alexithymia. Our emotions serve as a driving force and a compass in many situations. Biologically speaking, we show anger because we want others to be afraid of us. Sadness, particularly when accompanied by tears, shows that we are in need of help. We show pride because we expect the environment to praise us. This feeling can also amplify a positive collective feeling in a whole group. All our emotions serve as signals to the environment, and at the same time, they are driving the forces behind our own acts. Nature has different intentions associated with different emotions. Every emotion has both bodily and psychological expressions. When we clearly recognise an angry feeling in ourselves, we act differently compared to when we feel sadness. The first feeling may stimulate us to act with determined force. The second feeling may stimulate us to withdraw and become passive. For the most part, our acts will be adequate in relation to the emotion that we experience. Human beings (as well as many animals) develop a repertoire of feelings that we can identify and differentiate between. This repertoire gives us guidance in stressful situations. A person who has good skills in differentiating feelings is also likely to be able to differentiate

T. Theorell, *Psychological Health Effects of Musical Experiences*,
SpringerBriefs in Psychology, DOI: 10.1007/978-94-017-8920-2_9,

feelings in relatives, friends and family members. Accordingly, emotional competence relates to social competence. Like the development of all kinds of skills, it is likely that training in emotional skill should start as soon as possible in life. In psychosomatic medicine, inability to differentiate feelings is labelled alexithymia. Alexithymia is associated with increased risk of illness. The most well-documented example is hypertension (high blood pressure), which arises more often in alexithymic persons than in others (Grabe et al. 2010).

So how early should we start? Probably already at the embryonic stage! During the later part of the pregnancy, the embryo has fairly good hearing already, and it is able to differentiate sounds (Granier-Deferre et al. 2011). It has also been shown that the embryo can learn to differentiate vowels that are audible for it during this part of the pregnancy—the newborn child shows physiological signs (sucking behaviour) indicating that it recognises the mother's speech sounds from the foetus period (Moon et al. 2013). An American newborn child recognises typical American speech sounds, while a Swedish child recognises typical Swedish speech sounds. Speech melody—so-called prosody—is close to music for the child!

It could be assumed that the embryo's emotional experiences in the uterus are primitive. It is likely to recognise some aspects of the mother's movements, ranging from no movement at all to slow and fast, and from chaotic to rhythmic. In some way, the embryo may associate some movements with audible speech and music. The chemical environment may also change in association with these components of sensory input. It is a fact that some stress hormones, for instance cortisol, passes the placenta barrier. In other words, when the mother is stressed, joyful or sad, the chemical situation for the child will correspond to those maternal conditions. Other kinds of auditive stimuli may also play a role in this. For instance, the mother's heart sounds are audible to the foetus. In some way, the foetus may be able to differentiate between a fast motherly heart rate associated with fast bodily movements on one hand and a maternal tachycardia without bodily movements on the other hand?

Of course, when the child has been born, interaction with the environment becomes more intensive. The social anthropologist Dissanayake (2000) has performed detailed studies of the mother–infant interaction before the age of six months. Mimics, gestures, speech sounds and singing become important components of the emotional communication, particularly frequent with the mother.

During the first years after birth, the child develops an increasing ability to recognise different emotions and to differentiate between an increasing number of fine-grained emotional states. A child who gets no support in developing these skills will be handicapped not only as a child but potentially also later in adult years, because the emotional interpretation of important situations does not translate into appropriate actions—the core concept in alexithymia.

Music and other cultural experiences can help children in their emotional development, and here the concept multimodal is important. For instance, if one reads a legend to a child, music accompanying it may amplify the emotional context. This will facilitate for the child to identify the "correct" emotions and also to differentiate between sadness, anger and anxiety for instance. Rhythmic dance movements may further amplify the emotional expressions.

Many adult men have difficulties in differentiating sadness and anger—they may show anger when in fact they are sad. This results in many problems both in their families and in their workplaces. Among many women, there is a similar problem: When they get very angry, they are unable to show their anger and in an inadequate way instead start crying, giving the environment the "wrong signal". If these men and women had had a better support in their emotional education as children, might they not have less of these problems? A debated question relates to the "translation" of emotions into words. This may not be important. It is probably possible to "recognise correct feelings" without using words for them! That would require ability to relate feelings in the body to emotions, for instance.

A large ongoing study (Mosing et al. 2014; Theorell et al. 2014), based upon 8,000 participants aged 27–54 from the Swedish twin registry, has shown that there is a correlation between musical achievement on one hand and emotional competence on the other hand (assessed by means of an internationally widely used standardised alexithymia questionnaire). Compared with those who had the highest achievement in musical ability, professionals those who had never played (or sung) have significantly worse scores for emotional competence. In addition, there is a significant relationship between amount of musical practice on the one hand and emotional competence on the other hand; the more musical practice the participant had had throughout life, the better the emotional competence. It should be pointed out, however, that musical ability, amount of music training and emotional competence are all intercorrelated and they are all partly determined genetically. Genes seem to determine (Ullén et al. 2014) around 50 % of musicality (depending on which musical ability; rhythm, pitch or melody). Interestingly, of the three components in musicality ("melody", "pitch" and "rhythm"), ability to differentiate different levels of pitch is the least genetically determined. About one-third of alexithymia is genetically determined. Most of the relationship between number of musical practice hours and emotional competence seems to be determined genetically. Still, there seems to be good reason to believe that musical training can influence emotional competence.

Cognitive Ability

The role that early music training may have in a child's *cognitive* development (mainly mathematics and language) has been discussed intensively during later years. There are extensive studies showing that children who start playing an instrument at an early age have better musical and cognitive ability than other children. Most of this research, however, has been based on so-called cross-sectional studies. This means that musical and cognitive ability has been assessed in adult years, in retrospect. Therefore, it is not known whether there is a causal role of the musical training. An argument is that children who start playing an instrument at an early age differ from other children already at the onset. According to this reasoning, it is not a coincidence that the child starts so early. Perhaps the child is more mathematically talented to begin with. This is a way of questioning the significance of the musical training itself. Such questions could also be posed regarding children who attend special music schools. There are three studies in which these difficulties have been dealt with (Schellenberg 2004; Costa Giomi 1999; Costa Giomi et al. 2001; Moreno et al. 2009, 2011).

Schellenberg followed 144 6-year oldsters whose cognitive abilities were assessed with the use of specially designed standardised methods. They were randomly allocated to four groups. In two of the groups, the children were given extra musical education (singing and piano playing, respectively). One group was trained in drama. These activities continued for a whole year. The fourth group had no extra training at all. Reassessment of cognitive ability after a year showed that the children who had received music training had had a statistically significant advantage in their cognitive ability compared to the other groups. Interestingly, the children who had been trained in the drama group had developed a better social ability than the other children. Perhaps not so surprising! Costa Giomi (1997) and Costa Giomi et al. (2001) have published a similar study of the effects of early piano playing on the development of general intelligence. A significant advantage was shown for the piano-playing children compared to the others. This advantage was attenuated when the groups were followed for three years. Moreno et al. (2009, 2011) have published a third study of a similar nature. Children were randomised to two experimental groups. The children in one group received musical training and the children in the other group training in painting. The training in both groups continued for six months. The children in the musical training group had a more pronounced increase in general intelligence than the children in the other group, but the difference failed to reach statistical significance. The total number of children, 32, in the Moreno study was relatively small, and this may contribute to the lack of statistical significance. In summary, the evidence is promising and future research will show how large the effects are. Schellenberg and Weiss (2013) have summarised this research.

The first study, using modern neurobiological technique, showing that brains of instrument players differ from other brains was performed on violin players. Advanced studies of the brain structures of piano players have also been performed. They have indicated that some parts of the brain have been stimulated by early training in piano playing. Bengtsson et al. (2005) have shown that brain areas involved in fine-grained motor skills (the so-called pyramid routes) have obtained a greater plasticity in piano players. This means that these parts of the brain have a better adaptability in musicians than in others. The differences between a musician's brain and other brains are not only confined to those areas of the brain that correspond to motor skills in the fingers. One has also observed differences, to the advantage of the musicians, in brain areas related to mathematics and language skills. Rhythm ability seems to be of particular relevance. Ullén et al. (2008) have shown that there is a strong relationship between general intelligence and ability to imitate rhythms. It should be cautioned, however, that a recent study of 27–54-year old twins in Sweden (Mosing et al. 2014) showed that the relationship between musical practice and general intelligence is mainly genetically determined.

Despite the results from the Swedish twin study, individual training effects of musical ability on general intelligence may still be important theoretically, but the

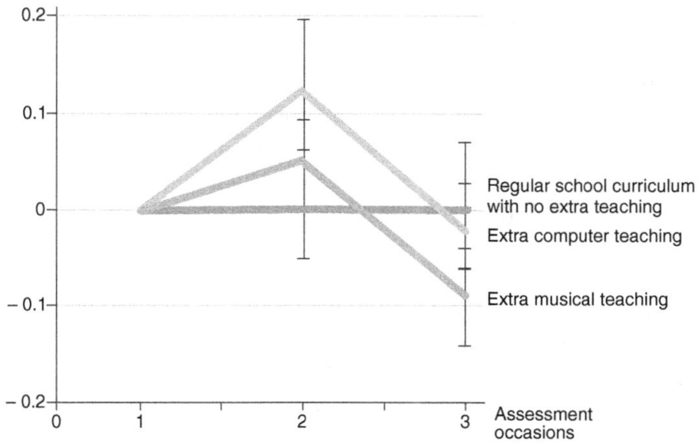

Fig. 9.1 Extra musical teaching and afternoon stress. Saliva cortisol concentration changes starting in August (with starting point equal to zero for all individuals) until December (2) and June (3) in three groups of children year 5–6 in schools in Stockholm. The points are based on logarithmically transformed averages of saliva cortisol concentration in the afternoon. The longitudinal lines with end points are equal to standard errors of means

effects of music training could only be established in large controlled intervention studies. Social mechanisms may also be of significance, however. Learning to play an instrument or to sing well may serve as an important focus in a life project for a child who has to organise his or her life in relation to it. It potentially gives a meaningful structure to the child's life. The effects of that could spread to other areas of life. It is important however that the training becomes joyful and associated with positive feelings. Otherwise, it may turn into something anxiety ridden that creates problems and inhibits learning. The best kind of music education in the school class could strengthen cohesiveness. This brings us back to the original use in man's history of music as an amplifier of cohesiveness.

A study that was performed by our group (Lindblad et al. 2007) in Stockholm originated in the old idea that music could be used as a means for strengthening the social climate in the classroom. There were three groups of pupils who were 11–13 years old during the study period. One of these groups had an extra music lesson lasting for 60 min once a week during the whole study year starting in August and ending in June the following year. The pedagogical idea was that the children would increase their awareness of one another and cooperate in the production of joyful sounds. This meant playful rhythmic songs and jingles, often with movements and with use of rhythmic instruments without demands for high musical achievement. The hypothesis was that the extra musical education would improve social climate and as a consequence of this also the learning environment. Two comparison groups of pupils of the same age were followed during the same study year; the first control group had the normal curriculum (which also included regular music teaching) without additions, while the second one had extra computer education once a week. Figure 9.1 shows how a biological measure of stress, the concentration of cortisol in saliva, developed during the study year. Changes in saliva cortisol mirror changes in blood cortisol. Since collection of saliva samples is painless and can easily be repeated, the assessment of saliva cortisol is often preferred to assessment of blood plasma cortisol. In this case, we were particularly interested in the afternoon assessments, when the pupils were likely to be more disturbed by a stressful classroom environment than in the morning. In the diagram, every individual pupil's starting value in the afternoon at the beginning of the semester in mid-August serves as reference point (=0). Mean changes in saliva cortisol are then shown for the assessments in December and June (end of second semester). There was a significant decrease in afternoon saliva cortisol in the "extra music" group but not in the two other groups. In the group with the regular curriculum, there were no changes at all, while in the computer group, there even tended to be an increase in saliva cortisol in December. In June, the mean level of saliva cortisol in the computer group was back to the initial level. So the results showed that the music group was the only group with a statistically significant decrease in afternoon saliva cortisol, corresponding to lowered stress levels, during the study year. The study was performed on relatively small groups (altogether 51 children), and it therefore needs to be replicated on larger groups. A tentative conclusion however was that the extra music education may have created an improved social climate resulting in lowered afternoon saliva cortisol. An important observation is that these processes seem to take their time—there was no significant improvement of "stress level" after only one semester. If it is true that such education creates a better social climate, it is also likely that the educational environment will improve and as a consequence the children will learn more at school. This has actually been tested in a much larger experiment performed in Switzerland (Patry et al. 1993; Spychiger 2002). A study was performed engaging 52 classes in Switzerland, half of which were randomly allocated to the experimental group (extra music education, one hour per week based on the cohesiveness idea presented above) and half of them to a control group (no extra music education). The experiment lasted for three years during which both groups were followed with assessments of social climate and achievements. The results showed that the music classes developed better social climate than the comparison classes. An important question was whether the fact that there was a slight reduction in the number of lessons in mathematics and languages would result in poorer mathematics and language achievements in the music classes. The results indicated that if there was a difference, it was rather in the opposite direction.

Music's role could be regarded in two different ways. First of all, Maria Spychiger (one of the leading researchers in the team) has pointed out that the teachers in classes with troublesome disturbing pupils were sometimes forced to work with the atmosphere in the classroom before they could start their extra music lesson. That something joyful, making interesting sounds together, was about to happen was an argument for calming down the atmosphere. When the children then started making the sounds, they discovered one another in a new way and this contributed to a calmed down situation. The musical education could accordingly be used as an argument for both calming down and achieving cohesiveness.

Many educational experts have extended the discussion regarding musical education from the formalised music education that is normally practiced in the school's music room to music components also in other school subjects. There are examples in several pedagogical systems, for instance in Steiner education where songs, rhythms, jingles and dancing are used in conscious ways in mathematics and reading.

The conclusion is that there is substantial evidence that musical education—if it is good and particularly if it strengthens the cohesiveness in the classroom—can improve the children's emotional and social development and that it can contribute to an improved achievement in mathematics and language. So far, we cannot be sure regarding the "web of causation". Is it a direct effect of the musical training that results in improved learning, or is it an indirect one going through an improved social climate resulting in good learning environment? We can make similar questions regarding musical ability in children. Children who start learning to play an instrument at a young age will not only train their finger skills and their musical ability; they will also get involved in creating a meaningful framework and goal for their life. Perhaps this is the most important aspect?

On the other hand, it is important for parents to realise that aspirations shall be reasonable and achievable. Too high aspirations and extreme discipline may give rise to mental problems. And mental problems are common among professional musicians whose situation will be discussed in the next chapter.

References

Bengtsson, S. L., Nagy, Z., Skare, S., Forsman, L., Forssberg, H., Ullén, F. (2005). Extensive piano practicing has regionally specific effects on white matter development. *Nature Neuroscience*, *8*(9), 1148–1150 (epub 7 Aug 2005).

Costa-Giomi, E. (1997). The Mc Gill piano project: effects of piano instruction on children's cognitive abilities. In A. Gabrielsson (Ed.), *Third triennial conference of the European Society for the cognitive sciences of music Sid* (pp. 446–450), Uppsala University.

Costa-Giomi, E. (1999). The effects of three years of piano instruction on children's cognitive development. *Journal of Research in Music Education 47*, 198–212.

Costa-Giomi, E., Gilmour, R., Siddell, J., & Lefebvre, E. (2001). Absolute pitch, early musical instruction, and spatial abilities. *Annals of the New York Academy of Sciences, 930*, 394–396.

Dissanayake, E. (2000). Antecedents of the temporal arts in early mother-infant interaction. In N. L. Wallin, B. Merker & S. Brown (Eds.), *The origins of music*. Boston: MIT Press.

Grabe, H. J., Schwahn, C., Barnow, S., Spitzer, C., John, U., Freyberger, H. J., Schminke, U., Felix, S., & Völzke, H. (2010). Alexithymia, hypertension, and subclinical atherosclerosis in the general population. *Journal of Psychosomatic Research*, *68*(2), 139–147. doi:10.1016/j.jpsychores.2009.07.015 (epub 17 Nov 2009).

Granier-Deferre, C., Ribeiro, A., Jacquet, A. Y., & Bassereau, S. (2011). Near-term fetuses process temporal features of speech. *Developmental Science, 14*(2), 336–352.

Lindblad, F., Hogmark, Å., & Theorell, T. (2007). Music intervention for 5th and 6th graders—effects on development and cortisol secretion. *Stress and Health, 23*, 9–14.

Moon, C., Lagercrantz, H., & Kuhl, P. K. (2013). Language experienced in utero affects vowel perception after birth: A two-country study. *Acta Paediatrica*, *102*(2), 156–160. doi:10.1111/apa.12098 (epub 9 Jan 2013).

Moreno, S., Marques, C., Santos, A., Santos, M., Castro, S. L., & Besson, M. (2009). Musical training influences linguistic abilities in 8-year-old children: More evidence for brain plasticity. *Cerebral Cortex, 19*, 712–723.

Moreno, S., Bialystok, E., Barac, R., Schellenberg, E. G., Cepeda, N. J., & Chau, T. (2011). Short-term music training enhances verbal intelligence and executive function. *Psychological Science, 22*, 1425–1433.

Mosing, M. A., Pedersen, N. L., & Ullén, F. (2014). Music training, music aptitude and IQ—Causality or genetic pleiotropy? A twin study. Manuscript. Department of Neuroscience, Karolinska Institute, Stockholm.

Patry, J.-L., Weber, E. W., & Spychiger, M. (Eds.) (1993). Musik macht Schule. Bericht and Schweizerischen Nationalfonds über den Schulversuch "Bessere Bildung mit mehr Musik". Freiburg/Ch.: Pädagogisches Institut der Universität.

Schellenberg, E. G. (2004). Music lessons enhance IG. *Psychological Science, 15*, 511–514.

Schellenberg, E. G., & Weiss, M. W. (2013). Music and cognitive abilities. In D. Deutsch (Ed.), *The Psychology of Music* (pp. 499–550). London, UK: Academic Press.

Spychiger, M. (2002). Music education is important—why? In G. Matell & T. Theorell (Ed.), *Stressforskningsrapporter*. Stockholm: Institute for Stress Research.

Theorell, T., Mosing, M. A., Lennartsson, A.-K., & Theorell, T. (2014). Musical activity and emotional competence—A twin study. Manuscript. Department of Neuroscience, Karolinska Institute, Stockholm.

Ullén, F., Forsman, L., Blom, O., Karabanov, A., & Madison, G. (2008). Intelligence and variability in a simple timing task share neural substrates in the prefrontal white matter. *Journal of Neuroscience, 28*(16), 4238–4243.

Ullén, F., Mosing, M. A., Holm, L., Eriksson, H., & Madison, G. (2014). Psychometric properties and heritability of a new online test for musicality, the Swedish Musical Discrimination Test. *Personality and Individual Differences, 63*, 87–93.

Chapter 10
The Musician's Health: To Earn One's Living from Music

If music has the potential of being beneficial to health, musicians ought to be more healthy than other people. No, this is not self-evident and musicians as a group are not extremely healthy. To earn one's living from music performances is not the same thing as playing for one's own joy. A career as a musician is not necessarily the amusing life that many non-professionals would believe. To be a symphony orchestra musician, participating in the performance of Beethoven's ninth symphony after having done this already one hundred and forty-seven times is not like doing it the first time. The same thing can be said about other pieces of music. Neurobiological research has shown that the professional musician uses his or her left brain hemisphere when listening to music much more than the non-professional person. This has been assumed to be due to the fact that the left brain hemisphere (in right-handed persons; in left-handed person this is reversed) is responsible for skills (in music listening, structures closely related to speech for instance) and "conscious" cognitive analysis. While the naive listener interprets the music more holistically (with activation mainly of the relevant structures in the right brain hemisphere), the professional will activate the corresponding structures on the left side at the same time. This illustrates that music changes meaning when a person goes through professional training. The skill-related interpretation "takes over" some of the emotional and holistic interpretation. In neurobiological research, it has been possible to show that professional music training changes the brain activation patterns and that these changes are progressive; singers who are training on conservatory level have more such changes in their brains than laymen and highly accomplished opera singers have more of them than the conservatory students (Kleber et al. 2010). One of my scientific collaborators who has had a career as a professional musician has told me that her experience of music changed completely when she stopped earning her living from music performances. Nowadays, her attitude to music is much more relaxed than it was during the professional years. This means that it is possible to "de-programme" some of the professional brain activation patterns.

What has been discussed extensively in relation to professional music making is performance anxiety. The professional musician perceives extreme expectations

T. Theorell, *Psychological Health Effects of Musical Experiences*, SpringerBriefs in Psychology, DOI: 10.1007/978-94-017-8920-2_10,

from the audience. This means that anxiety in the most demanding situations can be an overwhelming problem. In our days, this is amplified by the hard competition that characterises the music market. There are many professional musicians and few jobs. This creates strong competition with many negative effects. When I listen to conversations among musicians, I am sometimes reminded of frequently described problems in sports. For example, there are internationally famous singers who need to medicate in order to be able to perform on their world-class level. The extent of medicine use is not known since musicians and singers frequently do not want to admit that they use such medicines. Some of these medicines decrease tachycardia and inhibit finger tremor (both of which could disturb the performance), while others amplify normal stress reactions. The latter example may surprise, but exogenous administration of cortisone (which is very similar to the body's own cortisol) could be practiced by singers. The reason is that cortisone (and the body's own cortisol) dampens swollening of mucous membranes including those on the vocal cords. Accordingly, cortisone may make it possible to perform despite an ongoing cold or any tendency to swollening (caused for instance by overuse of the cords). This may be beneficial if it happens infrequently. However, if it happens frequently, it is risky for two reasons: First of all the same risks as those we associate with long-lasting stress reactions could arise if cortisone is used frequently in large dosages. Secondly, there is a risk that the musician will be increasingly biologically and psychologically addicted. This could mean that the body stops having the normal acute stress reaction before and during performances.

The "price of fame" in terms of reduced longevity among top stars in rock and pop has been described in a population study by Bellis et al. (2007) showing both in Europe and the United States that from 3 to 25 years "post-fame", the age- and gender-standardised mortality were almost doubled in this group compared with the general population.

For the soloist, performance anxiety is a real threat (see below. For those playing in a group or orchestra or singing in professional choir, some of the main problems during musical performances are more related, however, to the interaction with other musicians. Joy and satisfaction protects against the adverse effects. In a study of 250 musicians in twelve Swedish symphony orchestras (Liljeholm and Theorell 2003), it was shown that those who were satisfied with the conductor, the rehearsals and the choice of repertoire were more healthy (both mentally and with regard to the musculoskeletal functions) than other symphony orchestra musicians. This was true regardless of gender and type of musician (string or wind instrument). Accordingly, conditions related to the artistic satisfaction are the most important explanatory factors in relation to health. The professional musician who experiences satisfying musical productions is likely to carry this with him or her into everyday life outside the music arena as well!

What makes the situation so special for musicians and singers compared to the conditions in other occupations? The "routine" argument (about the decreasing joy associated with playing the same piece many times) could of course be applied to any occupation. Therefore, it is important to reflect upon factors making the musician's occupation special. One of the first factors coming to one's mind is that a musician who is part of a group, for instance an orchestra, depends to a higher degree on his or her colleagues than do those working in other occupations. The orchestra musician who commits an error during a rehearsal may force the whole orchestra to repeat. In two different studies, we have shown that orchestra musicians perceive their possibility to influence their own work situation as less than employees in most other occupations. Somebody else has decided what the orchestra should play and the conductor makes the immediate decisions regarding tempo, intensity and subtle shifts of the music's character. The individual musician may actually influence the total planning of year, the order of performances (the musicians may for instance want demanding productions to be followed by less demanding, etc.) through the programme committee in which the union takes part. But this is frequently not perceived as "real" influence. Most musicians seem to accept things as they are.

Symphony orchestra musicians have participated in many systematic health examinations. Important factors behind stress-related symptoms among them are (when this group is compared to other occupations) the relatively high work demands and the little influence and poor social support that they experience. Female musicians seem to be more exposed to these factors than male musicians (Holst et al. 2012; Liljeholm et al. 2003; Theorell et al. 1990). In our own studies, we found one group with an equally poor level of decision authority, namely subway train drivers. This seems logical since a subway driver has a tunnel and rails, a book of rules and a time table to stick to, and improvisation is almost impossible. Most of the symphony musician's conditions are determined by somebody else: choice of music, tempo, nuances, etc. Those at risk seem to illustrate the iso-strain situation described in the literature about work places with poor psychosocial working conditions (high demands, low control and poor support, Karasek and Theorell 1990). Muscle tensions that are related to primitive defence mechanisms such as wrinkling forehead, sitting at edge of chair and contract muscles in shoulders and neck are typical in this group. Figure 10.1 shows the prevalence of this type of muscle tension in men working in different kinds of occupations (Theorell et al. 1990). In this study, each individual was asked to rate the amount of such muscle "defence" tensions. The scores were summed up for each individual, and the means of these sum scores were compared across the occupations. Figure 10.1 shows that the orchestra musicians had much more muscle tensions than others. This is probably related to the high degree of concentration required during a rehearsal or concert. As soon as somebody commits an error, there is a risk that the whole orchestra will have to repeat the passage. The other members of the orchestra may become irritated because of the mistake. This is not the case when an office worker writes an erroneous letter on his or her computer. Most of the time he or she simply corrects the error and nobody will ever see that an error was committed. A finding with similar connotations is that the orchestra musicians tend to have a higher diastolic blood pressure during their ordinary work days (with rehearsals) than do subjects in most other occupations (Theorell et al. 1990). The diastolic blood pressure is assumed to mirror the degree of contraction in the small arteries in the periphery—which in its turn mirrors psychological tension.

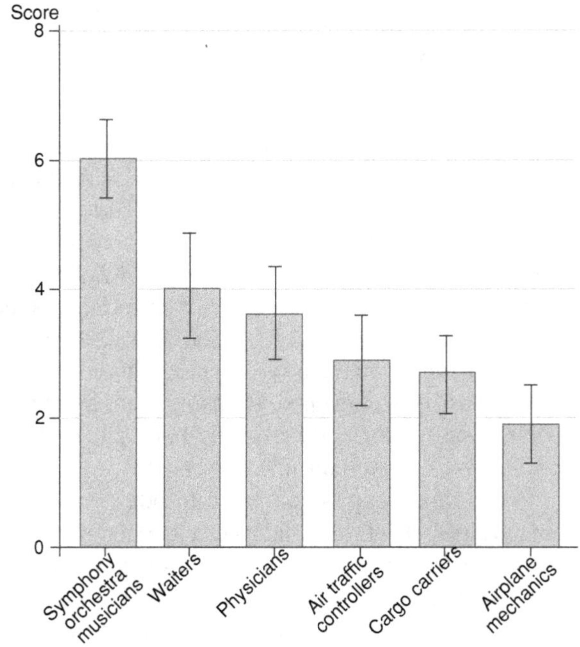

Fig. 10.1 Average muscle tension scores in different occupations (men). Mean score for muscle tension (possible range 0–22) in different occupational groups. The *longitudinal lines* with end point are equal to standard errors of means

The orchestra musicians depend on one another. Openness to advice from colleagues as well as their support in difficult situations contribute significantly and substantially to mental health in the orchestra studies (Holst et al. 2012; Liljeholm 2003; Theorell et al. 1990)—the better the support from colleagues the better the mental health. As soon as the social interaction is threatened by something that takes place in the orchestra, there will also be effects on the health of the orchestra members. This was illustrated in another study (Theorell et al. 2007) of two orchestras that we studied every 6 months during 2 years. In one of these two orchestras, a dramatic event occurred when the study was about to start—a wind instrument player fainted in front of audiences on two occasions during public performance. Both these concerts had to be interrupted. The other members became afraid that the same thing might happen to themselves and social tensions again arose in the orchestra. After some months, the situation calmed down when the musician stopped fainting (he received a pacemaker). The hormonal measure that was described in the stress chapter and in the chapter on choir singing, saliva testosterone, turned out to be very sensitive to this situation. The testosterone concentration in saliva showed a pronounced decrease in this orchestra and increased again when the stressor disappeared (see Fig. 10.2). Since saliva testosterone mirrors the regeneration activity, this potentially has great importance for healing and health development. When social cohesion is threatened, the biology is affected.

A striking feature in findings on the relationship between the orchestra's work environment and the health of their members is the importance of self-esteem.

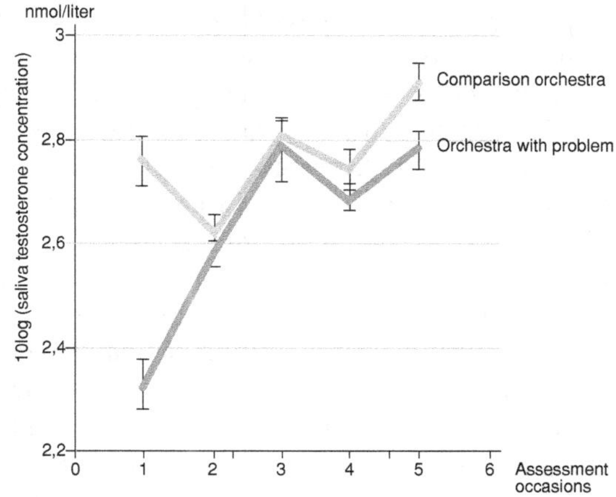

Fig. 10.2 Saliva testosterone in symphony orchestra musicians. The saliva concentration of testosterone has been assessed in two orchestras once every 6 months. In the orchestra with problems, the first assessment was made during the weeks after a musician had fainted on two different occasions in front of the audience. The *longitudinal lines*' end points are equal to standard errors of means

Those who play professionally in orchestras—particularly those with permanent positions—have been carefully selected in several steps. Difficult tests precede acceptance to the music colleges. When the musician has received his/her education, it is difficult to find a job in a professional symphony orchestra. Many spend several years (and even their whole professional life) as freelancers. This means short-lasting tasks one after the other in different orchestras. To obtain a permanent position is even more difficult. To reach that level one has to pass through several stages of tests, first an audition in front of orchestra members and then temporary employment during a test period. Those who rise to the level of leader of an instrument group have gone through these kinds of tests and test periods many times. They are often perceived as humiliating and anxiety provoking. Despite the fact that those who have a permanent position in a symphony orchestra have managed to go through all of this, they still complain that they feel insecure and not convinced that they are good enough (Liljeholm 2003). Female musicians have more problems with this than male musicians.

Stage fright has been the subject of several scientific studies (see for instance Fredrikson and Gunnarsson 1992). The basic problem is that the sympathetic nervous system is activated excessively, to a degree that is out of proportion to the situation. A certain degree of activation is desirable, but it should not be uncontrolled. One consequence of a strong sympathetic activation is hand tremor, making it very difficult to play a string instrument. Another common biological consequence is profused hand sweating—also preventing smooth execution of difficult passages since the instrument becomes slippery. For the singer, the problem may be a dry mouth and throat. Stage fright of such intensity that it creates a problem has a prevalence of around 15 % among musicians.

Performance anxiety (a wider concept than stage fright) is indeed a problem for many musicians and singers. This may in some cases have to do with childhood experiences. The musician who has been regarded as "talented" and "clever" in making music, all his/her life may have been severely criticised on all occasions when the performance has been less well. A furious perfectionism dealing with small details tends to make the whole existence "blue". For young people intending to start a career as a musician, this may lead to abandonment of such plans. For those musicians who have managed to get through in their career, stage fright is not diminishing with the years. When old age is approaching and the ability to withstand anxiety decreases, it may become impossible to continue a musician's career. New therapeutic techniques are developing, however, so there is help to be received. Psychological therapies are effective in many cases. Some medicines can be used effectively, if with caution and restriction. For instance, medicines blocking the beta-receptors in the sympathetic nervous system (beta blockers) can be used for string musicians who suffer from tremor during stage fright.

The possibility to handle stage fright is better in young age than in older. How stage fright functions in young age has been illustrated by a study performed by a group of psychologists (Fredrikson et al. 1992). The study was performed on second-year students at the Royal College of Music in Stockholm. They were about to go through their examinations. The examination consisted of a music performance that they had to do in front of a jury. Their performance was rated and this was part of their final grades. Heart rate and urinary excretion of adrenaline were biological measures of stress. They were also asked to rate how nervous they felt. Part of the performance was done anonymously without audience (the performance was taped and nobody knew who was playing when the tape was switched on), part of it openly with the teachers sitting in front of them looking at them during the performance. The anonymous and open parts were performed in random order. The results showed that those students who felt the highest degree of nervousness (and also showed more biological evidence of stress) were more disadvantaged by the open situation (compared to the anonymous one) than their fellow students. In the nervous category, the students had much better ratings when ratings were made anonymously. So even when they played objectively very well, their ratings were lower. Their nervous appearance obviously affected their ratings adversely. Accordingly, how the musician looks while performing could determine grades—to signal nervousness is a handicap even when the performance is good. How childhood experiences have an impact on nervousness could be illustrated by my own experiences. When I grew up both my parents were skilful instrumentalists and we were sometimes playing chamber music together. But I often felt insecure and when we had to repeat playing part of a piece because I had made a mistake, I always felt that my parents looked irritated and bothered. Pronounced performance anxiety has accompanied me when I have been playing the violin in front of an audience ever since. Later I discovered another kind of music making that was not as emotionally charged from my childhood, namely choir singing and singing in a group. Although I felt nervous on the first occasions when I was to sing a solo, the performance anxiety has been much less pronounced with singing than playing the violin.

That professionals have a different way of handling and listening to music does not prevent musicians from having very strong experiences during music performances—everything in music is not professional attitude even for the professional! In his book Beethoven's Anvil, Benzon (2001) writes about two famous musicians who have had strong experiences—trance states or changed consciousness—when everything worked very nicely during a performance in front of an audience. One of them was Leonard Bernstein who had such an experience when he conducted a symphony by Mozart. He experienced that he "was" Mozart and that he composed the music when he was standing there conducting. When the symphony was finished, others had to help him return to reality. The other one was Charlie Parker. When he was performing a saxophone solo in front of an audience, he experienced that he sat there looking at this person (Charlie Parker) who played. So musicians may also have strong and completely unexpected experiences when they perform music.

Finally, hearing problems are of course of particular importance for anybody who is making a living from music. Animal research (Tahera et al. 2006a, b) has shown that at least in mice exposure to stress with long-lasting increase in cortisol excretion (to the blood and to the brain) increases the risk that loud noise leads to permanent (rather than temporary) hearing loss. Mice who had been badly treated as newborn and young exhibited disturbed cortisol regulation (mainly with elevated levels). When they were exposed to noise they risked permanently impaired hearing. Mice who had had a "nice childhood" also showed evidence of hearing loss after noise exposure, but this loss soon disappeared. A recent study based upon a large number of subjects who had been asked to fill in a questionnaire regarding emotional exhaustion may illustrate that this may have relevance also for human beings (Hasson et al. 2013). Participants who had low ("normal") and high ("emotionally exhausted") scores, respectively, in the population study were asked to take part as contrast groups in an experimental study. In the laboratory, their hearing as well as the threshold at which they became unable to tolerate different kinds of sounds was assessed. This was done before and after they became exposed to acute stress in the laboratory. The results showed that the groups had similar hearing characteristics, including noise tolerance, before acute stress. After acute stress, participants in the exhausted group (particularly the women) had lowered noise tolerance whereas those in the normal group had increased their tolerance (had elevated their threshold). Accordingly, in normal conditions, we are able to "make ourselves" slightly deaf to noise when we are exposed to acute stress. But when we are emotionally exhausted we even become more sensitive to noise after acute stress. This may of course have profound relevance for musicians. A study (Hasson et al. 2009) showed that the hearing problems that symphony musicians suffer from become worse during some periods and that this is associated with a lowered activity in the stress-protective parasympathetic system (decreased heart rate variability, see the chapter on stress). There was also a tendency towards lowered saliva testosterone levels (reflecting lowered regenerative activity in general in the body) during periods with accentuated hearing problems. All these research findings point at complex interactions between long-lasting stress, acute stress and hearing problems. A musician who is constantly aroused and is not allowed to recuperate and relax between arousal periods will have an increased cortisol level in the body (including in the brain and the inner ear). That will make the risk of permanent hearing damage greater than in other musicians during exposure to strong sounds (of particular relevance for rock musicians who use strong amplification). And decreased regenerative/anabolic activity in the body (another consequence of long-lasting stress) may contribute further to this. The psychosocial work environment is accordingly of importance also in "hearing care".

References

Bellis, M. A., Hennell, T., Lushey, C., Hughes, K., Tocque, K., & Ashton, J. R. (2007). Elvis to Eminem: quantifying the price of fame through early mortality of European and North American rock and pop stars. *Journal of Epidemiology and Community Health, 61*, 896–901.

Benzon, W. (2001). *Beethoven's anvil: Music in mind and culture*. New York: Basic Books.

Fredrikson, M., & Gunnarsson, R. (1992). Psychobiology of stage fright: the effect of public performance on neuroendocrine, cardiovascular and subjective reactions. *Biological Psychology, 33*(1), 51–61.

Hasson, D., Theorell, T., Liljeholm-Johansson, Y., & Canlon, B. (2009). Psychosocial and physiological correlates of self-reported hearing problems in male and female musicians in symphony orchestras. *International Journal of Psychophysiology, 74*(2), 93–100. doi:10.1016/j.ijpsycho.2009.07.009 (epub 8 Aug 2009).

Hasson, D., Theorell, T., Bergquist, J., & Canlon, B. (2013). Acute stress induces hyperacusis in women with high levels of emotional exhaustion. *PLoS One, 8*(1), e52945. doi:10.1371/journal.pone.0052945 (epub 2 Jan 2013).

Holst, G. J., Paarup, H. M., & Baelum, J. (2012). A cross-sectional study of psychosocial work environment and stress in the Danish symphony orchestras. *International Archives of Occupational and Environmental Health, 85*(6), 639–649. doi:10.1007/s00420-011-0710-z (epub 20 Oct 2011).

Karasek, R. A., & Theorell, T. (1990). *Healthy work*. New York: Basic Books.

Kleber, B., Veit, R., Birbaumer, N., Gruzelier, L., & Lotze, M. (2010). The brain of opera singers: Experience-dependent changes in functional activation. *Cerebral Cortex, 20*, 1144–1152.

Johansson, Y. L., & Theorell, T. (2003). Satisfaction with work task quality correlates with employee health. *Medical Problems of Performing Artists*, 141–149.

Tahera, Y., Meltser, I., Johansson, P., & Canlon, B. (2006a). Restraint stress modulates glucocorticoid receptors and nuclear factor kappa B in the cochlea. *NeuroReport, 17*(9), 879–882.

Tahera, Y., Meltser, I., Johansson, P., Bian, Z., Stierna, P., Hansson, A. C., et al. (2006b). NF-kappa B mediated glucocorticoid response in the inner ear after acoustic trauma. *Journal of Neuroscience Research, 83*(6), 1066–1076.

Theorell, T., Ahlberg-Hultén, G., Sigala, F., Perski, A., Söderholm, M., Kallner, A., et al. (1990). A psychosocial and biomedical comparison between men in six contrasting service occupations. *Work & Stress, 4*(1), 51–63.

Theorell, T., Liljeholm-Johansson, Y., Björk, H., & Ericson, M. (2007). Saliva testosterone and heart rate variability in the professional symphony orchestra after "public faintings" of an orchestra member. *Psychoneuroendocrinology, 32*, 660–668.

Chapter 11
Final Thoughts

One of the conclusions that could be drawn from this book is that artistic subjects should have a more prominent role at schools. Indeed, the founders of the pedagogical systems Reggio Emilia (Malaguzzi 1971) and Waldorf (Uhrmacher 1995) used arguments supporting this. The Reggio Emilia system arose after the Second World War and the period of fascism under Mussolini in Italy. The founder claimed that arts have the ability to strengthen our empathy. Therefore, a skilful use of the arts at school is likely to prevent violent acts and attitudes when the children grow up to become adults. And the founder of the Waldorf educational system argued that arts are more central to the education of small children at school than cognitive training. Several authors (see for instance Nobel 2001) have argued that our era is overemphasising cognitive learning and that it will never be possible to educate children to become well-functioning adults only by teaching mathematics and language. And besides from moral and ethical arguments, it is also clear (as described in the chapter on children) that learning to play an instrument or to sing stimulates cognitive development resulting in improved development of general intelligence in early childhood. If used in multimodal pedagogics, music and other forms of arts can stimulate the cognitive learning processes also in children who do not actively train these skills. As I have mentioned, there has been a discussion regarding stimulation of intelligence also in adults via the "Mozart effect". It is clear that good and stimulating music, if well selected for the situation and for the group, can stimulate motivation and focus in a challenging situation, but this does not prove permanent effects on intelligence.

However, it is becoming increasingly clear in the scientific debate that emotional and social skills are just as important as cognitive ones. Emotions are our driving forces; those who are able to correctly interpret their own feelings in a challenging situation are also the ones who will be able to act in the most purposeful ways. This pertains to all kinds of feelings, anger, fear, sadness, joy, etc. Those who suffer from alexithymia (inability to differentiate between different kinds of feelings) run the risk of becoming confused because they wrongly interpret emotional signals from the environment. This is where music enters the picture

T. Theorell, *Psychological Health Effects of Musical Experiences*,
SpringerBriefs in Psychology, DOI: 10.1007/978-94-017-8920-2_11,

because music is such a useful tool in amplifying and inducing emotions as well as in helping to "translate" emotional processes.

The demand on scientists to establish "independent effects" is behind some of the difficulties that a researcher interested in music and health encounters. Is it the music "per se" that has effects on biological and psychological conditions? Music is always performed and consumed in a context, and therefore, it is very difficult to disentangle the musical effects from other environmental influences. I have myself been educated scientifically in a natural science framework and I consider it important to establish relationships by means of statistics and objective methodology. In societal planning, such knowledge is necessary. At the same time, however, we must remember that unique personal experiences are very real and could be extremely important. If many people have such experiences, the importance becomes profound. But they are often difficult to describe with the use of objective methods and statistics. They may "drown" when they are grouped in simple "countable" categories. A good example of this is the large collection of "strong musical experiences" tales reported by Gabrielsson (2011). These stories show that individuals may have experienced a completely new type of content in their lives as a consequence of one single musical experience—their total life changed. Such processes cannot be described by means of statistics. The question is how strong individual experiences should be valued? In a highly "developed" society, they should be highly valued, I think. A society with a rich and multifaceted musical life is a society which gives its members unique and fantastic musical experiences. My own country has been an example of this. There has been extensive musical education available for all children and youngsters at a low cost and with a solid basis in municipalities. Church-based music has been and is still very important for a vital musical life in our society. Many different forms of music have been stimulated. Emphasis on diversity is important since the stimulating effects can arise in any form of music if there are sufficient numbers of active performers and sufficient resources. It is often claimed that the classical music as well as church music are threatened in modern society. These are prophecies that have turned out to be wrong previously and are likely to be erroneous also today. If we have a sufficient number of engaged young people who are willing to learn how to perform high-quality music, we will always see the birth of new combinations of old and new music. This can be observed at the folk music festivals with participants from many countries.

An important prerequisite for a vital musical life in a society is a sufficient number of good professionals who can stimulate others. This requires a good and solid basis of musical education. It is important not to cut down music at school and in "culture schools" offering music education after school hours. Such a decrease would lead us astray in many ways. I have emphasised the importance of music during childhood and youth in preventing the fostering of a large group socially and emotionally incompetent adults, with alexithymia, which is a difficult social handicap. Public health would be negatively affected by such a development. It is important to offer our children a broad repertoire of musical experiences so that they have a varied musical background that they can relate to. This will make it easier for them to have a rich music life later in life. With increasing age, it is increasingly difficult to "conquer new domains", although it is never too late as the stories told by Gabrielsson tell us.

Even in the final stage of our lives, music may become very important. In the US, there is a movement called "Living Will", working for improved quality of life during the final stage before death. One of the prominent representatives of this movement, Donna Chadwick, who is a music therapist, has stated that all human beings shall get the opportunity to work out together with somebody else a list of pieces of music that should be played in the final stage, before death, when one is unable to talk or incapacitated to the extent that it is impossible to express preferences. The "somebody else" should preferably be a music therapist who has a deep and broad knowledge about different music styles and is able to interview the person about preferences and possible music repertoire. This list of music pieces should then be stored in such a way that it can be found when the situation arises (Chadwick and Wacks 2005). Many thoughts arise. Of course, it would be fantastic to get hospital staff to play my preferred music when death is approaching!

In this book, I have tried to describe how "good" musical activities can create calmer and better learning environments at school and how they can amplify and improve the effects of other pedagogical techniques. But of course, music can also, if used in adequate ways, be very important in private life and at work. The only problem is that the effects of music, like the effects of other cultural activities, are hard to predict. Sometimes, the effects may turn out to be negative. Music has been used as an amplifier of fanatic political messages and torture. Wrong music in the wrong place can give rise to strong negative feelings. This makes it very important to devote considerable energy to research on psychological and biological effects of different kinds of music. Development of this knowledge will make it easier to understand when and under what circumstances different kinds of music will do good and when it will hurt.

Björkvold (2005) has discussed pedagogical methods in music education. In line with many other authors (for instance Uddén 2001), he finds that traditional music education has overemphasised the cognitive aspects (training ability to read music, manage difficult passages, etc.) and that there is insufficient emphasis on joyful playing and improvisation. For instance, an important question is when a child should start learning to read notes. There is a conflict between the trained capacity to read notes on one hand and the ability to improvise and "play" in the music. I belong to the category of amateur musicians who became accustomed to reading notes. Accordingly learning by heart was not so important in music for me. Unfortunately, the note reading inhibits the ability to improvise and play in music. It may also reduce the tendency to get "carried away" emotionally by the music. But at the same time, I would never have had access to all the fantastic experiences of classical music (including many experiences of flow) without learning how to read notes. A balance between these modes of relating to music has to be reached.

As in other areas of cultural activity, research on biological effects of music has not started until fairly recently. I have described a few small efforts that I have been involved in myself and some of these throw light on the question why we feel good sometimes when we sing. One finding is that the concentration of oxytocin (which reduces anxiety and pain) increases during singing and also during listening to music under some circumstances. However, this hormone is only one in large group of hormones that are involved in the immediate biological reactions to music. In another study, we found that the excretion of one of the hormones involved in regeneration increased markedly when subjects started to sing in a choir. This points at a possible mechanism underlying health-promoting effects of regularly practiced singing. It relates to the body's ability to protect itself against adverse effects of stress by repairing and restoring worn-out cells. Our research also indicates that the training of singing ability stimulates the coordination between lung and heart functions.

On an international scale, music research is rapidly expanding, and in the near future, we shall have many more answers to difficult questions!

References

Björkvold, J.-R. (2005). *Den musiska människan*. Malmö: Runa Förlag.

Chadwick, D., & Wacks, K. (2005). Music choices for later life: The Advance Music Directive. Föreläsning vid den tolfte världskongressen i musikterapi, Brisbane.

Gabrielsson, A. (2011). *Strong experiences with music—music is much more than just music*. Oxford: Oxford University Press.

Malaguzzi, L. (1971). *Esperienze per una nuova scuola dell'infanzia—Atti del seminario di studio tenuto a Reggio Emilia il 18-19-20 marzo, 1971*, a cura di Loris, Editori riuniti.

Nobel, A. (2001). Om konst och eget skapande i undervisning (On art and creativity in teaching) Carlsson Bokförlag, Stockholm.

Uddén, B (2001). Musisk pedagogik med kunskapande barn. Vad Fröbel visste om visan som tolkande medel i barndomens studiedialog. (What Fröbel knew about folklore as an interpretative aid in childhood education dialogue) Centrum för musikpedagogisk forskning, KMH-förlaget, Stockholm.

Uhrmacher, P. B. (1995). Uncommon schooling. A historical look at Rudolf Steiner, anthroposophy, and Waldorf Education. *Curriculum Inquiry, 25*(4), 381–406. doi:10.2307/1180016.JSTOR1180016.

CPSIA information can be obtained
at www.ICGtesting.com
Printed in the USA
LVHW080836171121
703569LV00004B/118